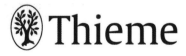

Tests and Exercises for the Spine

Peter Fischer, MTC, MSPT, DPT

Lecturer, Faculty of Medicine of the
University of Tübingen;
Private Practice
Tübingen, Germany

296 illustrations

Thieme
Stuttgart · New York · Delhi · Rio de Janeiro

Library of Congress Cataloging-in-Publication Data

Fischer, Peter (Physical therapist), author.
  [Tests und Übungen für die Wirbelsäule. English]
  Tests and exercises for the spine / Peter Fischer ;
  translator, Getrud Champe.
     p. ; cm.
  This book is an authorized translation of the German edition
titled Tests und Übungen für die Wirbelsäule, published 2012
by Georg Thieme Verlag, Stuttgart.
  Includes bibliographical references.
  ISBN 978-3-13-176001-2 (paperback) –
  ISBN 978-3-13-176011-1 (eISBN)
  I. Title.
  [DNLM: 1. Spine. 2. Exercise Test–methods.
3. Exercise Therapy–methods. 4. Posture. WE 725]
  RD771.B217
  617.5'64062–dc23   2014046026

This book is an authorized translation of the German
edition published and copyrighted 2012 by Georg Thieme
Verlag, Stuttgart. Title of the German edition:
Tests und Übungen für die Wirbelsäule

Translator: Getrud Champe, Surry, Maine, USA

Illustrator: Malgorzata & Piotr Gusta, Paris
Photos: Oskar Vogl, Affalterbach, Germany

© 2015 Georg Thieme Verlag KG
Thieme Publishers Stuttgart
Rüdigerstrasse 14, 70469 Stuttgart, Germany
+49 [0]711 8931 421, customerservice@thieme.de

Thieme Publishers New York
333 Seventh Avenue, New York, NY 10001, USA
+1-800-782-3488, customerservice@thieme.com

Thieme Publishers Delhi
A-12, Second Floor, Sector-2, Noida-201301
Uttar Pradesh, India
+91 120 45 566 00, customerservice@thieme.in

Thieme Publishers Rio de Janeiro, Thieme Publicações Ltda.
Argentina Building, 16th floor, Ala A, 228 Praia do Botafogo,
Rio de Janeiro 22250-040 Brazil
+55 21 3736-3631

Cover design: Thieme Publishing Group
Typesetting by Ziegler und Müller,
Kirchentellinsfurt, Germany

Printed in Germany by Aprinta GmbH, Wemding   5 4 3 2 1

ISBN 978-3-13-176001-2

Also available as an e-book:
eISBN 978-3-13-176011-1

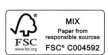

Important note: Medicine is an ever-changing science undergoing continual development. Research and clinical experience are continually expanding our knowledge, in particular our knowledge of proper treatment and drug therapy. Insofar as this book mentions any dosage or application, readers may rest assured that the authors, editors, and publishers have made every effort to ensure that such references are in accordance with **the state of knowledge at the time of production of the book.**

Nevertheless, this does not involve, imply, or express any guarantee or responsibility on the part of the publishers in respect to any dosage instructions and forms of applications stated in the book. **Every user is requested to examine carefully** the manufacturers' leaflets accompanying each drug and to check, if necessary in consultation with a physician or specialist, whether the dosage schedules mentioned therein or the contraindications stated by the manufacturers differ from the statements made in the present book. Such examination is particularly important with drugs that are either rarely used or have been newly released on the market. Every dosage schedule or every form of application used is entirely at the user's own risk and responsibility. The authors and publishers request every user to report to the publishers any discrepancies or inaccuracies noticed. If errors in this work are found after publication, errata will be posted at www.thieme.com on the product description page.

Some of the product names, patents, and registered designs referred to in this book are in fact registered trademarks or proprietary names even though specific reference to this fact is not always made in the text. Therefore, the appearance of a name without designation as proprietary is not to be construed as a representation by the publisher that it is in the public domain.

Contents

Contents

Contents

Contents

Preface

Currently available exercise books are lacking clear, test-based guidelines for the design of an efficacious, preventive, safe, and independent exercise program. These books only offer a multitude of exercises without any guidance on how these exercises can be meaningfully used. But "meaningful" does not mean doing any hundred exercises; it means doing the three that really help. It is also meaningful to select exercises not only because they ease the symptoms in the short term, but also because they eliminate the causes of the symptoms (e.g., a bad posture). This is the only way to exercise the spine into a healthy state and keep it fit.

So that this goal can be achieved time efficiently and with ease, I have developed the following spinal fitness check on the basis of 25 years of clinical and scientific work experience in physical therapy, both in Germany and the United States.

I wish you a healthy spine, great success in treatment and prevention, and, last but not least, fun.

Peter Fischer, MTC, MSPT, DPT

About the Author

After completing German Physical Therapy School in 1986, Peter Fischer moved to San Francisco, California, where he worked as a physical therapist in the outpatient clinic of the University of California San Francisco Medical Center and earned his MSPT and DPT degrees.

His research interest was identifying the qualities that a healthy spine requires and how these qualities may be acquired. In order to simplify spinal diagnosis and therapy, he has developed various instruments that are now sold worldwide: PALM (Palpation Meter, www.spineproducts.com), Posture Trainer (www.posture-trainer.com), and the diagnosis and exercise concept of this book (www.spinal-fitness.com).

In 1998, Peter Fischer opened a clinic in Germany specializing in the treatment of the temporomandibular joint, head, and spine. His practice team consists of 15 physical therapists. Definition of the treatment goals, monitoring of progress toward the goals, and communication of the results to the patient and the referring physician are part of his practice quality management.

Peter Fischer teaches the scientific basis and practice of physical therapy for the Faculty of Medicine of the University of Tübingen, Germany. His teaching duties for the university include the improvement and maintenance of spinal fitness for students, physicians, and staff. He provides the same services internationally for companies, public employers, schools, and sports teams, using the methods shown in this book.

In addition, Peter Fisher teaches the "Spinal Fitness Check" for the German Physical Therapy Association. In this course, he instructs physical therapists on how to apply the lessons outlined in this book to both individual patients and groups. Aside from training in the clinical application of the tests and exercises, the course also covers relevant aspects of biomechanics, differential diagnosis, and professional communication. If you would like to organize a course, please email the author directly at fischer@praxis-f.de.

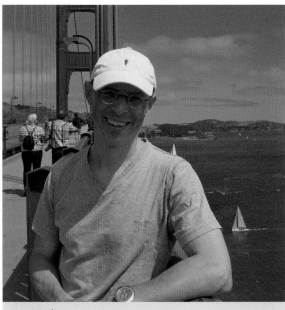

Peter Fischer

Essential Whys and Hows of Training and Testing

1 Why Exercises, Tests, Patient Language, and Navigator

In this book, you will find tests and exercises for posture, relaxation, movement, coordination, mobility, strength, and endurance, all of which are needed for a completely fit and healthy spine.

> **3 in 1**
>
> Diagnosis, treatment, and instructing the patient how to exercise independently can be carried out in one step. In addition, a navigation system indicates the right tests and exercises for any given area of symptoms and dysfunctions.

1.1 Why Do Exercises?

Exercises provide a more effective and lasting improvement for most functional disorders of the spine than does manual treatment alone. In addition, instructing a patient on how to eliminate a problem through exercise relieves the therapist, both physically and in terms of time management. One of the most frequent results of physical stress on the therapist is carpometacarpal joint arthritis. This results from our attempts to straighten or loosen something with our fingers that will be just as crooked and tight at the next appointment if the patient does not exercise. For this reason, the author nowadays uses manual techniques only for diagnosis and in those rare cases in which exercise alone is not enough (see Chapter 11).

> **Long-term efficacy**
>
> Therapists who work principally with exercises and only use manual techniques as a backup measure are more successful and have fewer symptoms themselves.

1.2 Why Perform Tests?

1.2.1 Efficacy

Every exercise in this book is preceded by a test that tells you whether or not the exercise is important for your patient. This distinction between important and unimportant exercises, allows for an effective and *time-efficient focus on the right exercises.*

1.2.2 Prevention

The tests help to find and correct weak points *before* they become apparent as pain and obvious impairment. This is considerably simpler and more efficacious than correcting weak points that have become so pronounced that symptoms have already developed.

1.2.3 Time Efficiency and Safety

The tests will also tell you when your patient has become adequately fit that she can decrease the frequency of an exercise or stop it altogether. This too saves time and *protects against injury resulting from excessive training* (e.g., instability caused by exaggerated mobility training or overloading through too much strength training).

1.2.4 Motivation and Responsibility

The tests let you see the progress that is being made through exercise. This visible success motivates the patient to keep on exercising. If the patient has not made any progress because she has not exercised, this will also become evident in the test and make it clear that improvement is needed in exercise discipline rather than in the therapist's choice of exercises. Thus, the test allows you to make the patient responsible for her own health: the success of the exercise plan depends on the patient's diligence in carrying it out. The therapist is required to reconsider his treatment plan only if the patient shows no improvement in her well-being or her function despite making significant progress toward a test goal.

> **First question**
>
> The first question to ask the patient should always be about exercise compliance. Only after you have an answer to this question does it make sense to ask whether her symptoms have changed.

1.2.5 Approval

The tests also increase diligence in exercising because your patient wants to make a good impression on you, knowing that the retest at the next appointment will show just how much or how little she has exercised.

1.3 Why Is the Exercise Always the Same as the Test?

When the exercise and the test are the same, the three tasks of "*diagnosis, treatment, and exercise plan*" can be carried out in one step. This saves time and ensures that the structure that has tested positive is exactly the one that will receive training. For instance, if the test for posterior thigh flexibility (p. 101) reveals insufficient flexibility, the treatment and home exercise program will consist of having the patient remain in the test position until the tension decreases. Regardless of whether the resistance is caused by muscle tension, connective tissue contracture, impaired neurodynamics, or a combination of these, this stretching exercise will always mobilize precisely those structures that are blocking the free mobility of the posterior thigh.

But if the diagnostic test and the treatment are not the same, the wrong structure might be treated. For instance, if the test for posterior thigh flexibility (p. 101) shows insufficient flexibility and the therapist suspects that the cause is impaired neurodynamic mobility in the intervertebral foramen between L5 and S1 and mobilizes this segment, he may be wrong. If the resistance is in fact a contracted ischiocrural muscle, his mobilization will have no effect.

1.4 Why Establish a Differential Diagnosis?

A differential diagnosis makes it possible to find the causes of a problem. This is a requirement for any efficacious treatment. Another important objective of differential diagnosis is to recognize whether a patient's symptoms are caused by a disease process that cannot be treated with physical therapy. In this case, the differential diagnosis allows us to refer the patient to a physician in the appropriate field, where she can be helped.

1.5 Why are the Tests and Exercises Written in Patient Language?

As opposed to all the remaining sections that are addressed to the therapist, the sections Test, Exercise, and Alternative Exercises are written in patient language. This distinction was made because the exact wording in patient instruction matters in reaching the objective of the test or exercise. The wording of the patient instructions presented in this book is based on years of everyday practical experience and the positive results of extensive monitoring, testing, and adaptation. The therapist may use this wording when directly addressing a patient or to bridge a short, unexpected break. A therapist who needs to take a call during treatment could ask the patient, for e.g., to "read and do this exercise within your range of comfort."

1.6 Why an Exercise Book with a Navigator?

The treatment navigator is an image of a human being in which individual body parts are numbered. If a patient presents with symptoms or dysfunctions in a specific area, the respective number directs the therapist to a series of tests and exercises that are most likely to detect and eliminate the cause of the respective symptoms or dysfunctions. The selection and order of the recommended tests and exercises are based on the author's 25 years of experience using the test and exercise system in this book. As in driving using a GPS, some people will be pleased with this orientation aid, whereas others would rather find their way alone.

2 Essential Training and Testing Q + As

• **How important are the following Q + As?**
The information in this chapter is essential for the safe and effective application of the tests and exercises in this book.

• **What is the difference between test and exercise?**
Almost none. The exercise is an attempt to pass the test.

• **Which exercises should your patient do?**
Only those exercises for which she cannot yet pass the test.

• **How often and how long should one do mobility, strength, and endurance exercises?**
  ◦ Mobility: once a day, until the tension relaxes and/or the mobility increases noticeably.
  ◦ Strength: three times a week until fatigue of the muscle group is sensed.
  ◦ Endurance: two or three times a week for 30 to 60 minutes.

• **How much extra time is required to practice good posture, relaxation, movement, and coordination?**
None. They should be a constant companion in everyday activities and become habitual.

• **How long should the daily practice of mobility, strength, and endurance exercises take, at most?**
Only a daily exercise program with a realistic time commitment has any chance of being followed regularly. To be realistic, the therapist should always ask the patient how many minutes a day she can picture herself exercising regularly and for the long term. The daily program should not take longer than that.

• **And if the test results recommend more mobility, strength, and endurance exercises than the patient is willing to do?**
If the patient does not have enough time or motivation to do all the mobility, strength, and endurance exercises for the test she was not able to pass, the therapist should decide which of these exercises are especially important.

Selection criteria

Two criteria for the importance of an exercise are (1) how far the patient is from achieving the test objective and (2) the degree of symptomatic relief that occurs immediately after completion of the exercise.

Another way to reduce the time spent on daily exercises is not to do all the selected mobility exercises every day but to divide them into two groups that are done on alternate days. Finally, many mobility, strength, and endurance exercises can be integrated into everyday activities without additional time expenditure. For instance, many exercises can be done while telephoning, watching television or standing in the elevator.

• **At what time of day should your patient exercise?**
It is a good idea to have a fixed exercise time, such as immediately on arising, before going to bed, or during the television news. Another possibility is to connect exercises to specific daily situations, for example "When I'm on the phone, I always lie down on my back and stretch the back of my thighs on the door frame."

• **When is your patient doing an exercise correctly?**
If she is getting closer to the test objective, for instance if she is becoming more mobile as a result of mobility exercises. In part, your patient will be able to feel this progress. However, for professional communication with the physician and patient, you should also document your patient's progress by entering the initial and subsequent test results in the treatment plan.

• **Which exercises are unnecessary?**
If your patient passes a test without having exercised, the corresponding exercise is not necessary.

Warnings and Contraindications

General warnings and contraindications are described under "Which exercises should your patient not do?" below. Make sure to read this entry along with the other Q + As of this section carefully before beginning with any of the tests or exercises in this book.
Specific warnings and contraindications are also found in various sections (e. g., "exercise" or "biomechanics") of the respective test or exercise. Therefore make sure to carefully read the entire chapter before the application of a test or exercise.

• **Which exercises should your patient not do?**
She should not do any exercises that her physician has advised her not to do or that cause or intensify her symptoms. If exercises cause or intensify symptoms, they should immediately be replaced by alternative exercises that do not cause any discomfort.
In cases of rheumatoid arthritis, Down syndrome, or long-term cortisone treatment, or after trauma to the cervical spine, such as whiplash trauma, you should first

ask your patient's orthopedist whether the chin tuck included in the following exercises is contraindicated: chin tuck mobility (p. 70), thoracic extension mobility (p. 73), hip flexion mobility (p. 95), buttock muscle flexibility (p. 96), and abdominal and anterior neck muscle strength (p. 117). In the case of pregnancy, disease, illness, trauma, or surgery, you should obtain permission from your patient's physician before beginning with any of the tests or exercises in this book.

- **How fit does your patient have to be in order to pass all the tests?**
  The tests are based on experience-based measures of posture, relaxation, movement, coordination, mobility, strength, and endurance that unlimited spinal function requires.

- **Should elderly individuals be expected to pass all the tests?**
  The fitness curves on page 194 clearly show how the progression from the "teens" (age 10–19) to the twenties (age 20–29) is associated with a significant loss of posture, relaxation, mobility, strength, and endurance. With the exception of a more pronounced loss of relaxation in women in their twenties, this development affects both sexes to the same extent. After this time, only men show a loss in fitness. From the age of 50, mobility and strength in men decreases.
  In the twenties, losses in fitness can be completely recouped through disciplined exercise. But as the bones and joints undergo degenerative changes with increasing age, passing all the mobility tests becomes less and less feasible. At this point, the treatment objective should be for the patient to decrease her distance from the test goals rather than to reach them. For instance, a 60-year-old patient who has not been training will hardly be able to regain the mobility she had when she was 20. But she could manage to regain the mobility she had 10 years ago. With the therapist's help, the frustration that some older patients experience when they see how much function they have lost should be transformed into motivation to "exercise their bodies 10 years younger," that is, to make the distance from the test goal (p. 179) a little smaller. Instead of aiming at the unreachable 100%, it makes more sense to show the patient the aging curve and to give her the goal of moving a decade to the left on this curve. If you direct your patients to this attainable 10-year goal and the corresponding standard, you will be able to motivate and reassure them.

- **How important is it to pass the tests?**
  It is not the most important thing for your patient to ever pass a test completely. It is more important for the tests to point to the correct selection of exercises by differentiating between relevant and irrelevant exercises. Depending on body type, previous injuries, surgery, or disease, it may even be impossible for the patient to

pass a certain test. Therefore, your patient should never use force while exercising but should gently move toward the test goal as far as is beneficial. Usually, the patient will already feel an improvement simply from getting a little closer to the goal. An overall guide to measuring your patient's progress toward the test goal is provided on page 179.

- **When can your patient reduce the frequency of or even stop the performance of an exercise?**
  - Posture, relaxation, movement, and coordination: These exercises should be carried out until they become habitual.
  - Mobility and strength: If exercising has made your patient fit enough to pass strength and mobility tests she could not previously pass, she should try to determine whether exercising less often is sufficient to maintain the strength or mobility she has achieved. To try this out, reduce the exercise by one session a week. As long as the patient continues to pass the test, the reduced exercise frequency is sufficient. If at some point a patient can pass the test without exercising at all, that exercise has become unnecessary and can be deleted from the program.

  If a deficiency is the result of age, continuous training will generally be necessary to maintain the strength and mobility regained through therapy. If the cause was only deficient posture, relaxation, movement, or coordination, correction of these aspects will make the corresponding strength or mobility exercises superfluous. With limitations due to surgery or injury, the outcome is less predictable, and time will tell whether and when the patient can decrease or stop certain exercises.
  - Endurance: Endurance training should be maintained for good.

- **In what order should your patient perform mobility, strength, and endurance exercises?**
  Ideally, in the following order: mobility, followed by strength, and finally endurance. Mobility exercises can be performed alone, but strength and endurance training should always be preceded by mobility exercises to prevent degenerative changes. If strength and endurance training causes undue muscle tightness, a follow-up with mobility exercises for relaxation may also be useful.

- **Which exercises are the most important?**
  For a healthy spine, it is most important for a patient to cultivate the right posture, relaxation, mobility, and coordination in the course of daily life. If these areas are in order, many symptoms will disappear spontaneously. If they are not, additional mobility, strength, and endurance exercises may be required. The most important of these is mobility, followed by strength, and finally endurance.

- **How do I know which exercises are right?**
  - If an initial test is passed, the patient should not be assigned the corresponding exercise.
  - If symptoms or dysfunctions have not improved even though the test goal has been achieved in the course of training, the corresponding exercise should be discontinued.
  - If the test has not been passed but the symptoms improve with the corresponding exercise, the exercise should be included in the exercise program and performed until the test is passed. When the symptoms have disappeared completely, no additional tests and exercises are necessary. If the test goal was achieved but the symptoms have not disappeared completely, continue with the next test in the selected Navigator (p. 146).
  - If an exercise is performed incorrectly, results in no progress toward the test goal, or cannot be performed at all, check the troubleshooting section for possible solutions. You can only determine whether the exercise is efficacious if it is performed correctly.

- **How soon should symptoms disappear with the right exercise?**
  If a mobility exercise is efficacious, the symptoms should disappear *immediately* after the improvement of mobility, that is, as soon as tension is relaxed while the body position is unchanged. The ability to perceive the relaxation and maintain the position does, however, require a certain amount of body awareness. In all other categories (posture, relaxation, movement, coordination, strength, and endurance), an effect should be noticed after at least 6 weeks of regular exercising. If no further compensatory mechanisms have set in and the exercises are done correctly, symptoms and functions may, however, improve spontaneously.

- **Why are all unilateral tests and exercises only described for the left side?**
  Tests and exercises that are performed individually for each side of the body are described for only one side (the left side) for reasons of brevity and clarity. Naturally, they are also to be performed analogously on the other side. For instance, if your patient passes one of these tests on the left side but does not pass it on the right side, she will need to do this exercise only on the right side.

- **What kind of equipment do you need for training?**
  Only things that are already there: a chair, a door frame, a free section of a wall or door, comfortable clothing, and a gym mat or blanket. For some exercises, a rolled-up towel or a cushion is also recommended. Finally, a mirror is helpful in learning the technique of abdominal breathing.

- **How can you determine whether your selection of exercises has been efficacious?**
  To determine how efficacious the exercises are, the therapist can document the patient's progress toward the test goals and the overall therapy goals (in terms of symptoms and function) in the treatment plan (p. 189).

- **How can you set up a professional exercise program for your patient?**
  When you visit www.spinal-fitness.com, you can download or printout a treatment plan for yourself and an exercise plan for your patient. You will find these downloads under "Information for therapists, trainers, and physicians." You can check off the exercises your patient should do on the exercise plan (p. 188).

Tests and Exercises
in Everyday Activities

3 Posture

3.1 Seated Posture with Symmetrical Foot Placement

Test

When you are seated, are your feet symmetrically positioned on the floor (**Fig. 3.1**) without one foot being further inside, outside, forward, or backward, or otherwise out of line (**Fig. 3.2**)?

Exercise

When you are seated, make sure that your feet are symmetrically placed (**Fig. 3.1**).

Troubleshooting

If symmetrical foot placement is not a daily habit, it may be the result of insufficient self-confidence, concentration, or mobility. Depending on the cause, possible solutions are as follows.

▶ **Self-confidence.** In some situations and social circles, crossed legs are considered elegant, casual, or demure. Make your patient understand how unstable and twisted crossed legs make the body, and how symmetrical foot placement and an upright posture radiate stability and poise. If this is unsuitable in some situations, asymmetrical foot placement should only be maintained for as long as necessary.

▶ **Concentration.** If symmetrical foot placement is not maintained from day to day because of distractions, reminder notes can be helpful at places where patients often catch themselves with an asymmetrical foot placement.

▶ **Mobility.** Asymmetrical foot placement can also be an unconscious attempt to compensate for unilateral tension or hypomobility. If this is the case, the tense or hypomobile tissues should be identified and mobilized with the help of the following tests and exercises:
- Posterior thigh flexibility (p. 101)
- Anterior thigh flexibility (p. 113)
- Inner thigh flexibility (p. 106)
- Buttock muscle flexibility (p. 96)
- Hip flexion mobility (p. 95)
- Calf flexibility (p. 103)
- Posture-friendly environment (p. 27)

> ### Alternating asymmetry
> Individuals who even after all these troubleshooting measures still do not feel comfortable without an asymmetrical foot placement should at least change sides every 5 minutes. If, for instance, the right foot is further forward, they should change after 5 minutes and advance the left foot.

Before and After Comparison

For what percentage of the day is the seated foot position symmetrical?

Differential Diagnosis

Possible causes of an asymmetrical foot placement that must be investigated can be found under "Troubleshooting" for this section. The patient often provides an indication of the causes of her asymmetrical foot placement when asked: "How do you feel in the corrected position?" If the patient reports that she feels tension in her hip joint in the symmetrical position, mobility in this area must be examined. If the patient says that symmetrical foot placement is impossible because, for example, a table leg is in the way on one side, this ergonomic impediment must obviously be eliminated. If the patient complains that she looks inelegant if she does not cross her legs, this mental block must be overcome. In this way, the simple question "How do you feel in the corrected position?" often provides decisive indications and is also worth asking for all the following posture exercises.

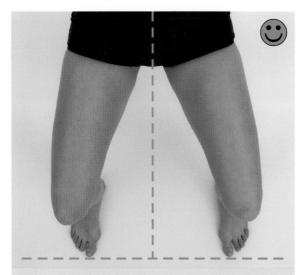

Fig. 3.1 Symmetrical foot placement.

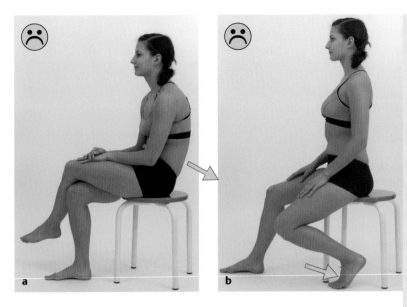

Fig. 3.2

a The most popular and damaging asymmetrical leg position: sitting with crossed legs leads to slouching and is often the cause of problems in the sacroiliac joint. Moreover, this position impedes venous return in the crossed leg and thus contributes to the formation of varicose veins.
b Asymmetrical leg placement with one foot under the chair.
c Pelvic rotation caused by asymmetrical hip abduction.

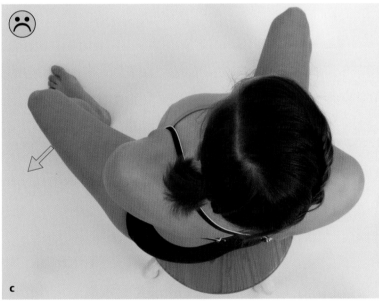

Biomechanics

Asymmetrical foot placement causes twisting and tension in the legs that is transmitted to the hip, pelvis, and spine. Conversely, symmetrical foot placement facilitates a neutral spinal curvature (p. 12) without twisting (p. 21). If this posture is consistently maintained during everyday activities, many posture-related problems disappear spontaneously.

3.2 Neutral Spinal Curvature

Test

Have you raised your sternum so far forward and upward that your spine is 75% erect while your head is loosely tipped forward so far that the front of your head is lower than the back of your head (compare **Figs. 3.3** and **3.4**)?

You can straighten your spine to 75% in the following way (**Fig. 3.5**). Start with a completely slouched posture (0% erect) and straighten yourself in four equal steps until your back is arched as far as it will go (100% erect). If you now release this posture by one step, you will be 75% erect and have found at your neutral spinal curvature (**Fig. 3.5 d**). In other words, the neutral spinal position is one step before your back is maximally arched.

Dynamic posture

The 75% erect position should not be rigidly maintained. Rather, it should be the midpoint of a dynamic posture (p. 53).

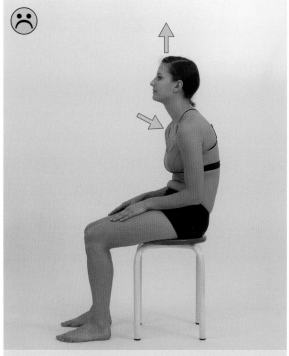

Fig. 3.3 Incorrect posture.

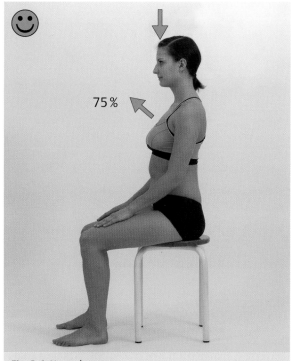

75%

Fig. 3.4 Neutral posture.

Exercise

Maintain a neutral spinal curvature with an average of 75% erectness, as often and for as long as is possible and comfortable.

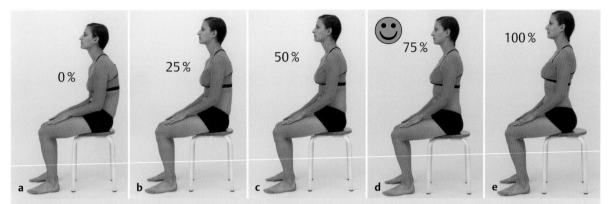

Fig. 3.5 Spinal straightening in four steps from completely slouched (0% erect) to where the back is arched as far as possible (100% erect).

▶ **Alternative exercises.** **Figs. 3.6** and **3.7** present images that can help in straightening your spine.

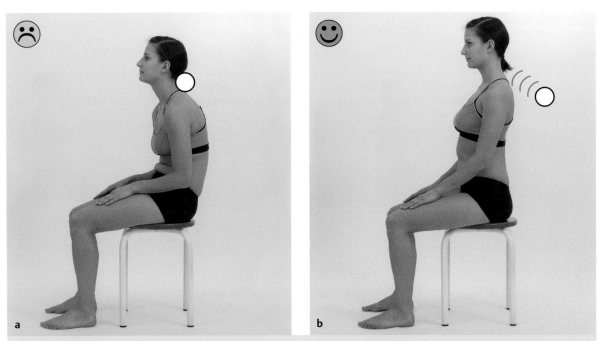

Fig. 3.6 Your slouched posture allows a ball to lodge at the back of your neck, where it exerts pressure and causes symptoms (**a**). Straighten up and imagine that you discard the ball (**b**).

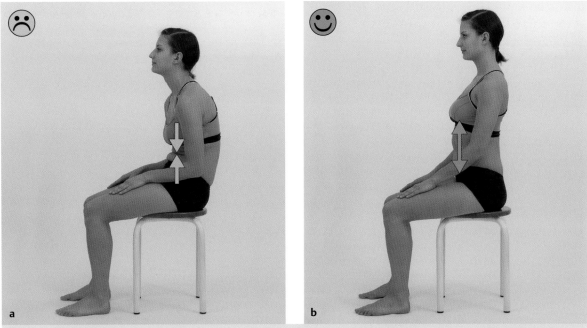

Fig. 3.7 Create a large distance between your rib cage and your pelvis, like a wide-open mouth. Feel how this increases the space for your heart, lungs and abdominal organs, so that these areas now feel lighter and more comfortable (**b**) than in the slouched posture (**a**).

Troubleshooting

If an erect posture is not a daily habit, it may be because of insufficient motivation, self-assurance, concentration, ergonomics, strength–endurance, or mobility.

Have your patients read this "Troubleshooting" section. They might see themselves in some of these points and then be able to apply the corresponding solutions.

▶ **Motivation.** Knowing the advantages of an erect posture is a source of motivation. Ask your therapist to explain the advantages to you. They are listed under "Biomechanics" for this section. Also learn how to replace a sense of obligation with a sense of pleasure by means of the following awareness exercise:

Awareness exercise: Well-being

Start with the question "How does the 75% erect posture feel compared with your usual posture?" Note that 90% of all individuals will first notice that the 75% erect posture requires more effort and is less pleasant than the old one. Now concentrate on where in her body the patient feels better in the 75% erect posture. Allow the time for her to find at least one such place. After initial doubt, everyone sooner or later succeeds in finding one. A typical sense of improvement in the 75% erect posture is the feeling of freedom in the abdomen, a better feeling in the lumbar spine or shoulders, or a lighter feeling in the neck. Let's assume that the latter is what the patient has recognized. Now the sense of pleasure can replace the sense of obligation. This means that instead of "I must persevere in this unpleasant posture because it is healthy," the patient can now tell herself: "I'm going to enjoy the feeling of lightness in my neck more often and liberate myself from the self-imposed imaginary ball lodged at the back of my neck (see **Fig. 3.6**)."

▶ **Self-confidence**

When your posture is erect, you radiate positive qualities —self-confidence, strength, readiness, fitness, balance, and poise.

Impression on others

Your posture affects how others see you.

But concerns that an erect posture might have negative implications will discourage anyone from assuming it. Typical and partly founded concerns of this kind are listed in the following awareness exercise "Fear."

Awareness exercise: Fear

Do you let the following fears keep you from maintaining an erect posture?

- My friends may not think I'm cool.
- I'm taller than most people, so I'll stand out or look different.
- I'll be a bigger target.
- The boys will stare at my breasts more.
- When I straighten up, I can't hide my big belly.
- I'll look stiff.

How can fears of this nature be addressed?

The spine should be erect but not stiff or rigid. It is easy to prevent an erect posture from looking stiff by means of dynamic posture (p. 53) and lively gestures and facial expression.

In the long run, an erect posture will usually cause the volume of the belly to decrease, because the intestines can work better in that position, with less bloating. In addition, more calories are burned as a result of the muscle work required to maintain an upright posture. Finally, a full stomach can be felt sooner in the upright position, which can serve as a feedback signal that the stomach is sufficiently filled.

This leaves the other points that cannot be as easily refuted. Solutions to these points require social intelligence. In most situations, it makes sense to replace negative sentiments with positive ones. For instance, instead of "With an erect posture, I will be a larger target," one can think: "Through my erect posture, I will radiate so much self-confidence and strength that no one will want to attack me." Or instead of "My friends may not think I'm cool if my posture is straighter," it's better to think: "I'll decide for myself what's cool!"

And even if there should be situations in which a slouching posture seems more advisable, it should not become a habit. Rather, it should be consciously replaced with an erect posture as soon as the situation has passed.

But what if upright posture does not suit the person's psychological mood? The mind–body connection is not a one-way street. This means that, on the one hand, our mood influences our bodily functions such as posture. Conversely, our mood can also be somewhat improved by a good posture.

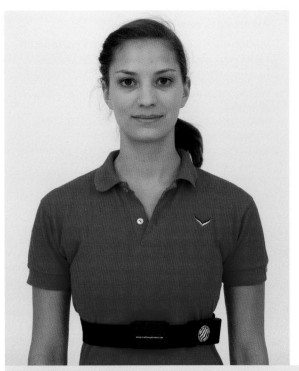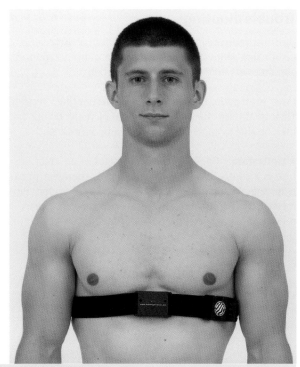

Fig. 3.8 The posture trainer.

▶ **Concentration.** If upright posture is not maintained in daily life because we become distracted and forget it, working with an automatic posture trainer can be useful (www.posture-trainer.com). The posture trainer (**Fig. 3.8**) saves the posture the user was in when the device was turned on as her threshold posture. It then vibrates until the user resumes a posture that is straighter than the threshold posture. A study with the posture trainer showed that the habitual thoracolumbar extension (erectness) while seated at the workplace is only 40% of the maximum available extension. With the automatic feedback, the thoracolumbar extension can be increased to 70% (www.posture-trainer.com — "Studies").

▶ **Ergonomics.** Often a person's surroundings, for example the configuration of their workplace or apartment, can make an upright posture impossible. Thus, eliminating these obstacles is much more useful than any manual therapy. Typically, it will take a physical therapist only 20 minutes to reconfigure the workplace to the patient's advantage.

In addition to adjusting the chair, desk, and computer, it is helpful to see whether the patient is using glasses with progressive lenses to work at a monitor. Since the reading portion of the progressive lens is usually located in the lower part of the glasses, the only position in which sharply focused near vision of a monitor at eye level is possible is with an unphysiological hyperextension of the cervical spine. The only solution for this problem is special computer glasses with a focal length corresponding to the distance between the eyes and the monitor. Naturally, this also applies to all other reading material in the near range that is not on the desk but vertically in front of the eyes, such as a musical score at eye level on a music stand.

Photo of the patient at work

If the physical therapist cannot visit patients in their workplace, they should bring him photographs or a video showing them at work.

▶ **Stamina.** There can be many reasons why an erect posture is initially experienced as strenuous. If the back muscles are atrophied as a result of slouching, they can be quickly rebuilt by switching to an erect posture. In spite of initial muscle soreness, an erect posture usually no longer seems strenuous after 3 to 4 weeks. An erect posture is the best training for the back muscles. It costs nothing, not even time, and trains the muscles precisely to the right extent. A study has shown that simply with posture training, the strength of the back extensors can be significantly improved in 6 weeks (Waibel et al 2013).

Erect without effort

From the start, the conversion from slouching to an erect posture is possible without a feeling of effort if the patient works with a dynamic posture (p. 53).

▶ **Mobility.** The erect posture becomes even easier when elastic resistance is relaxed. If one of the following tests is positive, an upright posture becomes easier immediately after doing the corresponding exercise:
- Chin tuck mobility (p. 70).
- Thoracic extension mobility (p. 73).
- Rotational mobility (p. 90)
- Posterior thigh flexibility (p. 101)

Before and After Comparison

For what percentage of the day is the spinal curvature neutral?

Differential Diagnosis

The following awareness exercise describes how you can test whether elastic resistance in the posterior thigh is impeding an erect posture.

Awareness exercise: Resistance

Sit on a table or a low wall in such a way that your legs can swing freely. If your knees bend when you switch from a slouched position to erect posture, you know that elastic resistance in your posterior thigh is making an upright posture more difficult.

The ideal seat for this test is a low wall or kitchen counter because your heel moving from dangling free (**Fig. 3.9a**) to hitting the wall or the base cabinet of the counter (**Fig. 3.9b**) will make you aware of any knee flexion taking place. In a slouching position (**Fig. 3.9a**), the heels should be two fingers width away from the wall or the base cabinet so that they can make contact in the upright position (**Fig. 3.9b**).

Biomechanics

A healthy spine requires an erect posture (Fischer 2004). Only when this posture is maintained consistently will the following posture-related problems improve permanently (**Fig. 3.10**).

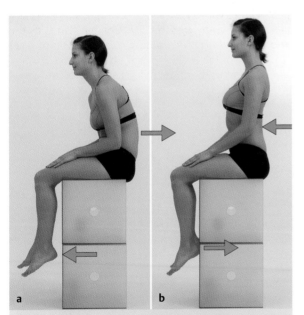

Fig. 3.9 Sitting on an elevated surface.

a Left: In the starting slouched position, the distance between the heels and a vertical surface should be two fingers in width.

b Right: If the ischiocrural muscles are too short, the knees bend automatically when the lumbar spine is in lordosis.

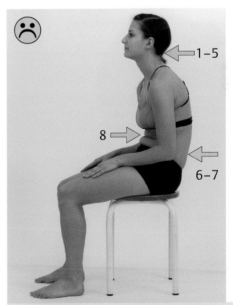

Fig. 3.10 Adverse effects of a slouched posture: (1) tight neck muscles, (2) blocked joints, (3) pinched nerves, (4) compressed disks, (5) less room for the spinal cord and vertebral artery, (6) stress on the intervertebral disks, (7) atrophied back muscles, and (8) compressed abdominal organs.

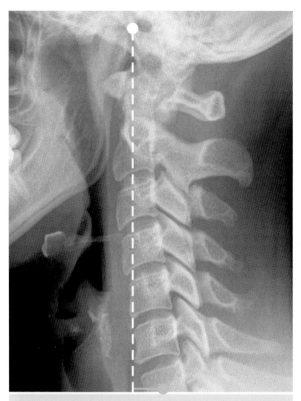

Fig. 3.11 Plumb line through the center of gravity of the head (white). Lever arm for the neck muscles (orange).

▶ **Tense neck muscles.** The lever arm (**Fig. 3.11**) for the neck muscles is shown by the horizontal line (orange) between the pivot point in the vertebral body of C7 and the plumb line (white) through the center of gravity of the head.

The torque that the neck muscles must counterbalance is equal to the weight of the head multiplied by the length of the lever arm. **Fig. 3.12** shows how a slouched posture lengthens the lever arm, requiring greater tension in the neck muscles to hold the head up.

If the head of an adult with an average head weight of 5 kg is displaced forward by 6 cm relative to the pivot point of C7 as a result of slouching, the torque is increased by 3 Nm. This explains why the myoelectric activity of the neck and shoulder muscles increases with a flexed posture (Schüldt et al 1986, Marshall et al 1995, Yoo et al 2006).

Tension in the neck muscles is also increased because slouching makes abdominal breathing more difficult, thus increasing the costosternal breathing component, with more tension in the cervical auxiliary breathing muscles.

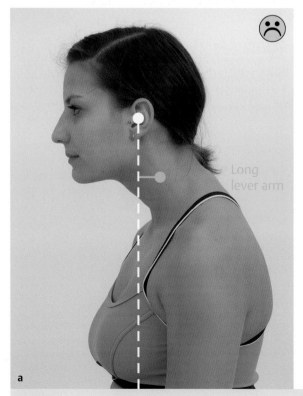

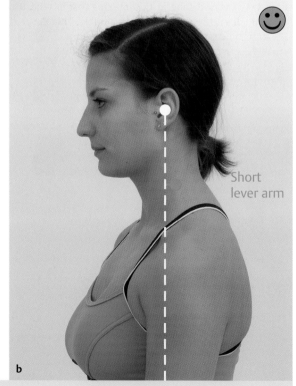

Long lever arm

Short lever arm

Fig. 3.12

a A long lever arm with a slouched posture and the head held forward (left).
b A short lever arm with an erect posture (right).

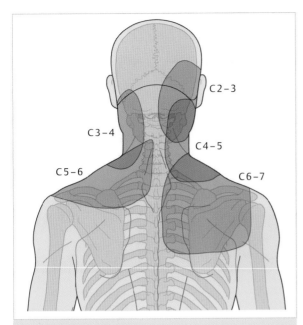

C 2 – 3

C 3 – 4

C 4 – 5

C 5 – 6

C 6 – 7

Fig. 3.13 Projected pain.

▶ **Blocked joints and pinched nerves.** A forward head position leads to increased extension of the middle and upper cervical spine. This hyperextended posture increases the compression of the facet joints and the emerging nerve roots (Farmer 1994). The pressure on the facet joints restricts mobility and leads to degenerative changes in these joints, which can restrict the emerging nerve roots even further.

> ### Awareness exercise: Ease of cervical rotation
>
> In a slouched position with your head displaced forward (see **Fig. 3.12 a**) as far as possible without discomfort, turn your head to one side and note what you can see at the outer limit of your visual field in this position. Now turn your head back to the middle and repeat this movement, but this time with a corrected posture (see **Fig. 3.12 b**). Feel how much easier it is and how your visual field has expanded with the corrected posture.

Overloading the facet joints by ventral displacement of the head may cause local or referred pain (Dwyer et al 1990, Kim et al 2005) (**Fig. 3.13**).

▶ **Pinched disk.** The forward position of the head that leads to increased extension of the middle and upper cervical spine compresses the posterior portion of the disks (**Fig. 3.14 a**). It is conceivable that this compression promotes pain, tears, and herniation in the posterior portion of the disk.

▶ **Less room for spinal cord and vertebral artery.** Extending the cervical spine narrows the spinal canal. This narrowing may compress and inhibit the neurodynamics of the spinal cord, especially if the spinal canal was narrow to start with. Cervical extension also reduces the lumen of the vertebral artery, while cervical spine flexion promotes symmetrical circulation in the common carotid arteries (Caro et al 1991).

If the transverse foramen is narrowed unilaterally, the blood flow to the brain may be reduced, but only if the circulation through the other arteries that supply the brain (both internal carotid arteries and the contralateral vertebral artery) is impaired. As long as the flow in only one artery is insufficient, the brain is still so well supplied by the other, unimpaired arteries that the patient usually remains symptom-free (Rivett et al 1999).

Neck muscle tension increases even more in the slouched position because it leads to ventral displacement of the head, thus overstretching the anterior neck tissue. The elastic tension of these tissues pulls the lower jaw backward and down. This downward pull must be counterbalanced by increased tone in the muscles that extend the neck and elevate or protrude the mandible. The elevated tone in the jaw muscles increases the tone in the neck extensors even more. This influence can be easily felt by patients lying on their backs if the therapist pushes his fingertips directly under the occiput into the neck extensors and asks the patient to protrude her lower jaw (see **Fig. 4.5**). The tension will now be distinctly greater than when the patient relaxes her lower jaw and lets it slide back toward the floor with gravity (see **Fig. 4.6**). The following awareness exercise can be used to show the patient how a head forward position interferes with the function of the cervical muscles.

> ### Awareness exercise: Muscle balance
>
> It can easily be felt how slouching with the head displaced forward (see **Fig. 3.12 a**) interferes with muscle balance if you try to swallow in this position. Then compare how much easier it is to swallow in the erect position (see **Fig. 3.4**).

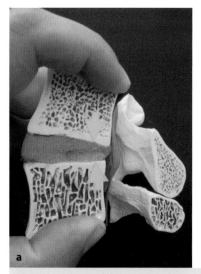
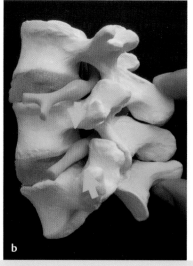
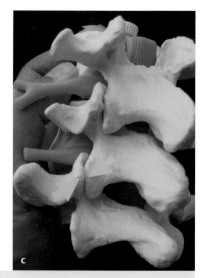

Fig. 3.14 Effects of end of range extension on the vertebral segment.

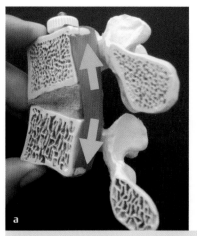
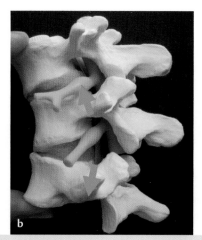
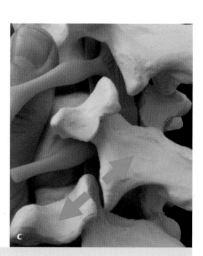

Fig. 3.15 Effects of end of range flexion on the vertebral segment.

▶ **Disk overloading.** If the back extensor muscles are deactivated by slouching, gravity flexes the lumbar and thoracic spinal segments to the point where they are held only by their connective tissue. In this case, the spinal tissues are compressed anterior to the axis of flexion and hyperextended posterior to the axis of flexion (**Fig. 3.15 a**).

Thus, the compression affects the anterior portion of the disks and the anterior part of the vertebral body. The bone of vertebral bodies is less dense (spongiosa = sponge-like) than the bone of the vertebral arch (compacta = compact). For this reason, habitual slouching over the course of the years leads to irreversible wedge-shaped deformation of the vertebral bodies that is clinically visible as kyphotic deformation.

Hyperextending the posterior tissues (the posterior portions of the disks, posterior longitudinal ligament, joint capsule, and interspinal ligament) for only 10 minutes decreases the stability of the spinal column (Little and Khalsa 2005). In addition, the disks are more intensely stressed in the slouched position since, in this posture, the facet joints do not carry any load (Adams and Hutton 1980, Nachemson 1981).

Kyphosis stress

At first, slouching feels comfortable to many people because the lumbar extensors are relaxed, the intervertebral foramina are wide, and the facet joints are not bearing a load. However, in the long term, this can damage the bones, disks, and ligaments.

▶ **Atrophied back muscles.** Habitual slouching causes the back extensors to atrophy. Thus, the muscular stability of the vertebrae and the iliosacral joints is lost. This adds stress to the joints, joint capsules, ligaments, and disks. Conversely, consistent posture training strengthens the back muscles, which can then often reposition and stabilize twisted vertebrae and iliosacral joints.

▶ **Compressed abdominal organs.** Slouching compresses the abdominal organs. In addition, it impedes free abdominal breathing, which—like a massage—improves the circulation, motility, and function of the abdominal organs. In addition to the liver, kidneys, gallbladder, and pancreas, it is particularly the stomach and intestines that profit from an erect posture and free abdominal breathing. Therefore it is worthwhile trying to find out whether digestive disorders improve with an erect posture. For instance, although a hiatal hernia will not close as the result of an upright posture, extending the spine reduces the pressure on the stomach and the likelihood that the stomach contents will be pushed through the hernia back into the esophagus. By reducing this backflow, an extended posture may help to ease the discomfort of reflux esophagitis.

3.3 Sitting without Side Bending or Twisting

Test

Are your pelvis, chest and head all facing in the same direction (**Figs. 3.16 b** and **3.17 b**), so that no part of your body is bent to the side or twisted? Check this in front of a mirror.

Exercise

When sitting, be sure your spine is not bent to the side or twisted.

▶ **Alternative exercise.** If you have persistent problems in the corrected position, you should ask your physical therapist to find the cause and suggest a suitable treatment or alternative posture.

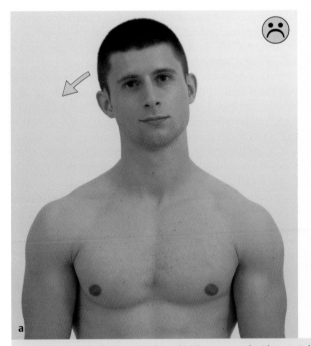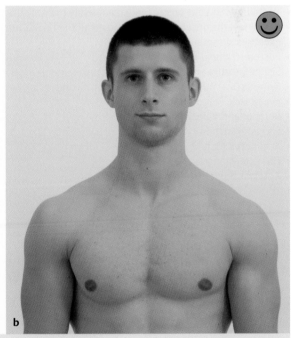

Fig. 3.16 Tipping the head to the side (**a**), compared with a straight head position (**b**).

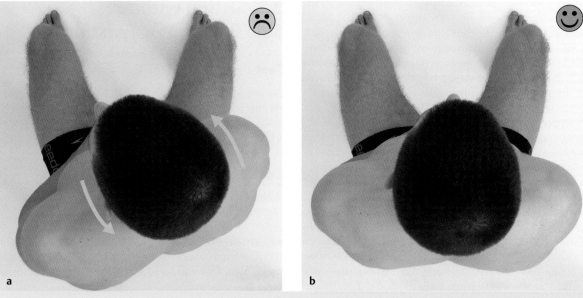

Fig. 3.17 A twisted upper body position (**a**) compared with an untwisted position, in which the upper body and the pelvis face in the same direction (**b**).

Troubleshooting

If the posture with spine untwisted causes persistent tension, seek out and resolve possible mechanical obstacles using the following tests and exercises. If one of the following tests is positive, have the patient do the corresponding exercise and determine whether this makes the untwisted posture possible without tension. If the answer is yes, you have found and resolved the blockade.

- Try to untwist your posture, not completely but only until you feel the onset of tension, and do all the relaxation exercises simultaneously (pp. 39–49)
- Posture-friendly environment (p. 27)
- Seated posture with symmetrical foot placement (p. 10)
- Symmetrical weight distribution when sitting (p. 30)
- Eye muscle coordination (p. 65)
- Rotational mobility (p. 90)
- Shoulder mobility (p. 78)
- Arm nerve mobility (p. 83)
- Hip extension mobility (p. 109)
- Anterior thigh flexibility (p. 113)

What to do in cases of scoliosis

If idiopathic scoliosis is present, complete correction cannot be expected. Correction should only proceed as far as possible and as long as it improves the patient's function and symptoms.

Before and After Comparison

For what percentage of the day is the spine positioned without side bending or twisting?

Differential Diagnosis

The most frequent causes of spinal twisting in the transverse (rotation) and frontal (side bending) planes are faulty ergonomics, scoliosis, habitual asymmetrical movement patterns, and unbalanced eye muscles. Scoliosis is expressed in the form of a rib prominence on the convex side of the scoliosis when the spine is flexed. The identification of ergonomic shortcomings and their elimination is described under "Posture-friendly Environment" (p. 27). With a little luck, habitually asymmetrical movement patterns can be detected in the course of a therapy session at the clinic. If this does not occur, ergonomic shortcomings and asymmetrical movement patterns can be best recognized if you visit and observe your patient in her workplace. If the asymmetrical movement pattern is a means of guarding or compensating, the area that is being guarded or compensated for will show by becoming symptomatic when you ask your patient to correct the asymmetry. A patient that keeps her head rotated to the right in order to compensate for a loss of hearing on the right side, for example, will hear less if she returns her head to a neutral position. Unbalanced eye muscles can often be detected and improved by means of the eye muscle coordination test and exercise (p. 65).

Biomechanics

An untwisted spine relieves the disks, joints, nerves, and muscles of the torques arising from a twisted posture.

A twisted spine is often caused by scoliosis. If the cause of the scoliosis is unknown, the scoliosis is termed *idiopathic.* In this most frequently occurring type of scoliosis, the vertebral bodies are deformed at the apex of the scoliotic curve. Especially after the termination of growth, the deformation of the vertebral bodies can no longer be corrected by physical therapy. However, even in such cases, partial improvement of the scoliotic curve is still possible through a correction of the corresponding deficits in posture, mobility, and strength.

Significance of the eyes

Disequilibrium of the eye muscles is offset by a rotation of the cervical spine. For instance, if the lateral rectus muscle of the right eye is contracted or hypertonic, the eye assumes a somewhat abducted position. This means that it "faces" somewhat to the right. In order to be able to look forward in spite of this, patients will typically compensate by keeping their head turned a little to the left.

3.4 Stabilized Neutral Spinal Curvature

Test

Can you maintain the natural hollow of your back and the unchanged chin to chest distance of a neutral spinal curvature when leaning forward and backward by moving only your hip joints and no other joints in your body (compare **Fig. 3.18 a–c**)?

To check this, first assume a posture with neutral spinal curvature (see **Fig. 3.4**).

Then spread the thumb and index finger of one hand as far as possible, place the index finger in the middle of your waistband or belt at the back and the thumb at the highest lumbar vertebra that you can reach (**Fig. 3.18**). As you lean forward and backward, try to keep the distance between your index finger and thumb, and thus the natural hollow of your back, unchanged (**Fig. 3.18**).

When you lean back, make sure that the distance between your index finger and thumb does not decrease. Conversely, when you lean forward, you should be particularly careful that the distance does not increase, and that the thumb does not slide downward on the spine.

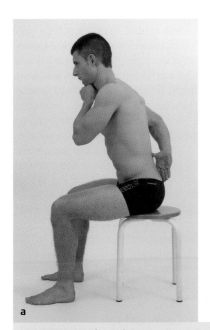
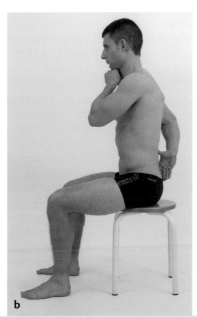
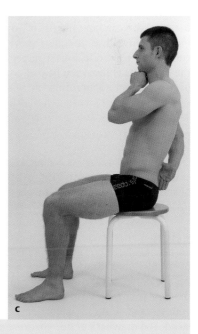

Fig. 3.18 Neutral spinal curvature.

a Leaning forward by flexing the hip.
b In an intermediate position.
c Leaning backward by extending the hip.

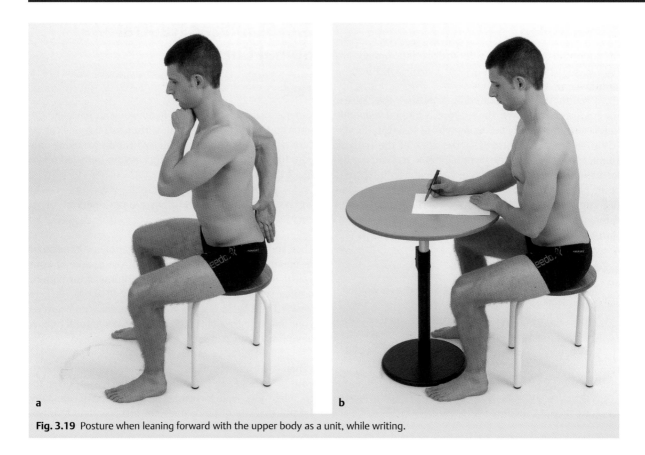

Fig. 3.19 Posture when leaning forward with the upper body as a unit, while writing.

Your chin to chest distance should also remain the same when you lean in either direction. To ensure that this is the case, you can hold the fist of your free hand tight to the sternum with your chin (**Fig. 3.18**). After some time, you will be able to lean your upper body as a unit from the hip joints without the help of your hand and use this posture at every opportunity in your everyday activities (**Fig. 3.19b**).

Exercise

During everyday activities when your spine is under particular mechanical stress (e.g., when lifting, pulling, or pushing), and when you are leaning forward or backward, be sure to maintain a stabilized neutral spinal curvature.

▶ **Alternative exercise.** If your shoulder mobility is limited, placing the thumb and index finger on your back in order to monitor the curvature of your lumbar spine might be uncomfortable or impossible. In this case, you may monitor your spinal curvature by placing your thumb on your sternum and your index finger on your abdomen instead. The drawback of this checking position is that you must determine whether a change in the distance between the two fingers is caused by respiratory movements or a change in spinal curvature.

Troubleshooting

If a patient cannot assume a neutral spinal curvature, suitable solutions are offered under "Neutral Spinal Curvature" (p. 12). If, on the other hand, leaning forward and backward from the hip joint is a problem, the following tests and exercises should be used to detect and resolve possible mechanical hindrances. If one of the following tests is positive, have your patient do the corresponding exercise and determine whether it then becomes possible to lean forward and backward from the hip joint more easily. If the answer is yes, you have found and resolved the blockade.

- Chair height (p. 28)
- Distance between the knees and between the feet while seated (p. 29)
- Seated posture with symmetrical foot placement (p. 10)
- Buttock muscle flexibility (p. 96)
- Posterior thigh flexibility (p. 101)
- Hip flexion mobility (p. 95)

Before and After Comparison

For what percentage of the day is a stabilized neutral spinal curvature maintained under stress (e.g., when lifting, pulling, or pushing) as well as when leaning backward and forward?

Differential Diagnosis

If the correct chair height (p. 28), a wide distance between the knees and between the feet while seated (p. 29), or symmetrical foot placement (p. 10) makes it easier to lean forward with a stabilized neutral spinal curvature, flexion at the hip joints was hindered by an unsuitable leg position. If leaning forward and backward improves after the buttock muscle flexibility (p. 96) or the posterior thigh flexibility (p. 101) exercise, the movement was blocked by insufficient flexibility in the corresponding region. Improvement by means of the hip flexion mobility exercise (p. 95) indicates insufficient flexion in the hip joint. Finally, patients with poor muscular stability of the lumbar spine will subconsciously tend to extend their lumbar spine in leaning backward and flex it in leaning forward.

Biomechanics

The stabilized neutral spinal curvature exercise (p. 23) makes it possible for the patient to maintain the protective neutral spinal curvature (p. 12) even under stress (e.g., when lifting, pulling, or pushing, or in a leaning posture). This short-term stabilization during exceptional stress has a strengthening effect and keeps the vertebrae in the right position. During extended activity without special stress, such as sitting at a computer, dynamic posture (p. 53) is important in order to avoid the strain of static posture.

3.5 Balanced Upper Body when Seated

Test

Is your upper body in a balanced position?

In order to find the answer to this question, first feel the tension in your abdominal muscles by pressing your fingers of your left hand slightly into your abdomen, just above the pubic bone (**Fig. 3.20 a**). If you do not find your pubic bone, press your fingers into your abdomen at the upper edge of the pubic hair. Place your right hand with the thumb pointing forward on the right iliac crest while the tips of the other fingers lie on the back extensor muscle on the right (**Fig. 3.20 b**) that lies close to your spine as a vertical muscle strand. If this is unpleasant for your right shoulder, switching sides is just as good (**Fig. 3.20 c**).

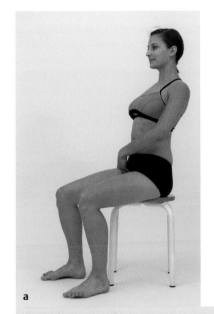
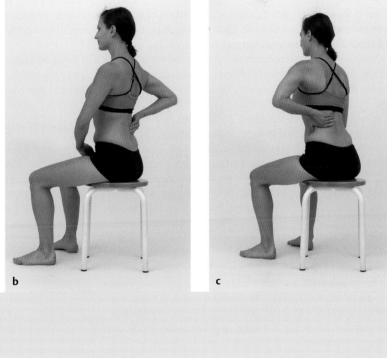

Fig. 3.20

a Upper body leaning backward.
b Upper body balanced.
c Upper body leaning forward.

If you now lean backward slightly from the vertical position with a stabilized neutral spinal curvature (p. 23) (**Fig. 3.20 a**), you can feel with your fingers how your abdominal muscles tense in front and push your fingers out of your abdomen while at the same time your back muscles relax.

In the same way, you can feel how your back muscles tense and your abdominal muscles relax as soon as you lean forward a little from the vertical position with a stabilized neutral spinal curvature (**Fig. 3.20 c**), as you would if you wanted to see more of your feet.

In the balanced position midway between leaning forward and leaning backward (**Fig. 3.20 b**) you can feel how back and abdominal muscles are equally relaxed.

Exercise

If you sit for long periods, make sure that your upper body remains close to vertical.

▶ **Alternative exercise.** Try to see whether you can feel the alternation between abdominal and back muscle tension when you lean backward and forward, even without using your fingers. This trains your body awareness and lets you find the balanced upper body position in every situation, quickly and inconspicuously. Soon this awareness exercise will teach you that the tension also changes in many other muscles when you lean forward or backward.

Troubleshooting

If the patient is not able to feel the alternation of muscle tension between the front and back muscle chains, check whether she has really placed her fingers on the erector spinae and rectus abdominis muscles. In very obese patients, the superior end of the rectus abdominis directly under the xiphoid process may be felt more easily than its inferior end. Moreover, alternation of the muscle tension will be distinctly felt only if the lordosis of the lumbar spine is maintained unchanged, as described under "Stabilized Neutral Spinal Curvature" (p. 23), while leaning forward and backward from the vertical. If the lordosis does not remain constant, the probing finger cannot distinguish between changes in muscle tension and changes in the spinal curvature. If the lumbar spine is not sufficiently lordotic, the erector spinae muscle does not tense sufficiently to produce a clear contrast between tension and relaxation.

If the patient remains rigidly in the vertical position, make her aware of the fact that the balanced position should be the midpoint of a dynamic posture (p. 53). In other words, one should cross the balanced position repeatedly but never stop midpoint, at that position. At the same time, the spine should never be away from it for long, in order to avoid excessive muscle tension. Most beneficial for the body are tiny, continuous movements around the midpoint of the balanced upper body posture with neutral spinal curvature. Examples of such movements can be found in the exercise on dynamic sitting and standing (pp. 53–56).

Before and After Comparison

For what percentage of long periods of sitting is the upper body close to vertical?

Differential Diagnosis

Many jobs require a *forward*-leaning upper body posture while sitting, creating increased tone in the dorsal muscle chain. Patients with tense back muscle, as a result of this type of working posture will report that the tension in this area increases in the course of a working day.

In contrast, a habitually *backward*-leaning upper body posture while sitting is usually not caused by working conditions. This overloads the anterior muscle chain from the anterior tibial, the iliopsoas, all the way up to the temporal muscle. As a result, symptoms can arise anywhere along this chain. For instance headaches can be caused by continuously elevated tone in the temporal muscle.

The most frequent cause of a habitually backward-leaning upper body is an extension deficit in the thoracic spine. In order to keep the line of sight level in spite of a thoracic hyperkyphosis, two means of compensation are typically applied. In addition to the frequently seen compensation by means of hyperextension of the cervical spine, the line of sight can also be raised by leaning backward. Usually, a mix of compensation mechanisms is used.

If habitual leaning back with the upper body causes symptoms, it is prudent to test, and if necessary also to improve, thoracic extension mobility (p. 73).

Biomechanics

With equal relaxation of the anterior and posterior muscle chains, the balanced upper body posture removes pressure from the disks and prevents early muscle tiring. Since the torque required to balance the trunk musculature in the balanced upper body position is approaching zero, an upright posture becomes an effortless matter. This makes the balanced upper body an ideal midpoint of dynamic posture.

3.6 Posture-friendly Environment

Test

Is everything that you frequently use (e.g., chair, table, computer keyboard) or look at (e.g., book, another person, computer, or TV screen) placed or set so that you can use it while sitting or standing with a neutral, balanced spine posture?

Exercise

Place everything that you frequently use or look at in such a way that you can use it sitting or standing with a neutral balanced spine posture (**Fig. 3.21**).

Troubleshooting

If suggestions for ergonomic solutions are not implemented or maintained, it is often because they are too inconvenient or too expensive, depend on someone else's approval, or require personal initiative.

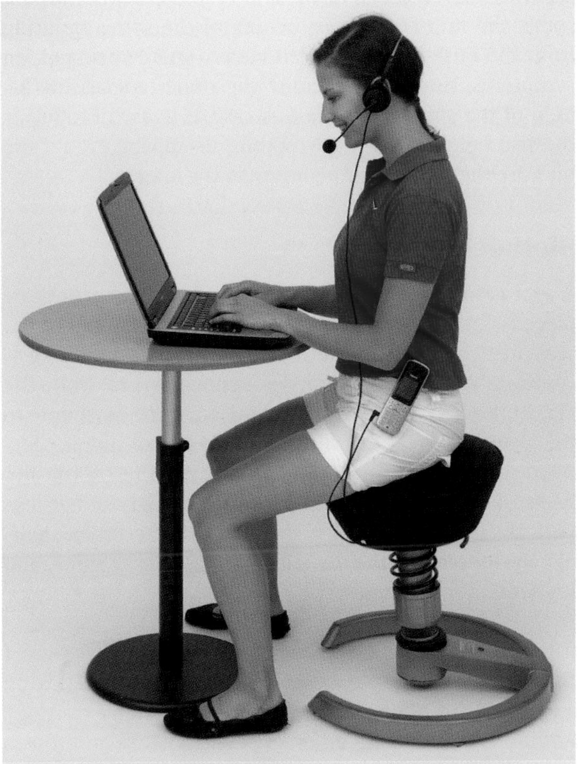

Fig. 3.21 An ergonomic workstation.

If, as a physical therapist providing ergonomic consultation for a company, you conclude that the company's management should buy new ergonomic furniture, equipment, or tools, it is advisable to discuss this first with the management rather than the employees. In this way, if the management rejects your suggestion, you avoid disappointing the employees and harming the workplace atmosphere.

The best solutions are the ones that you, as a therapist, put into practice yourself, on the spot and with the tools on hand. For this reason, it is advisable for you to have at least a screwdriver with exchangeable bits available, so that you can adjust desks, etc. If the desk and screen are not high enough, they can be set on the packages of copy paper that are available almost everywhere. In addition, it is helpful to have with you a little assortment of low-cost items, such as directions for exercises, lordosis supports, book rests, wrist supports, and a headset for the telephone, that you can if necessary lend or sell to your patient.

Standards

Never rely on ergonomic standards, such as a specific angle at which the arms or legs should be placed. The standard is a statistical average composed of a wide range of individual variation. Based on your qualifications and duty as a physical therapist, it is incumbent upon you not to force your patient into a standard mold but to recognize her individual biomechanical equilibrium and help her to find it.

Before and After Comparison

What percentage of your patient's day is spent in an ergonomically designed environment?

Differential Diagnosis

It is most effective to observe patients in the locations where their problems arise. For instance, if symptoms increase while a patient is working at the computer, observe her at her workplace and undertake the appropriate corrections on the spot. As a rule, 20 minutes at the workplace are time enough to do this.

If a visit to a workplace is not possible, a photo or video of your patient at work might be helpful in identifying the problem and finding the right solution. For example, your patient can ask a colleague to take a cell phone picture of her at work.

Biomechanics

The most important, basic biomechanical principles that an ergonomic environment should ensure are:
- A neutral joint position (pp. 10–38)
- Short lever arms (p. 18)
- A conscious release of unnecessary tensions (pp. 39–49)
- A dynamic posture and alternation between contraction and relaxation (pp. 50–57)

3.7 Chair Height

Test

Is the height of the chairs on which you regularly sit for extended periods high enough that your hips (**Fig. 3.22**, ①) are somewhat higher than your knees (**Fig. 3.22**, ②)?

Exercise

Make sure that the height of the chairs on which you regularly sit for extended periods is high enough that your hips (**Fig. 3.22**, ①) are somewhat higher than your knees (**Fig. 3.22**, ②).

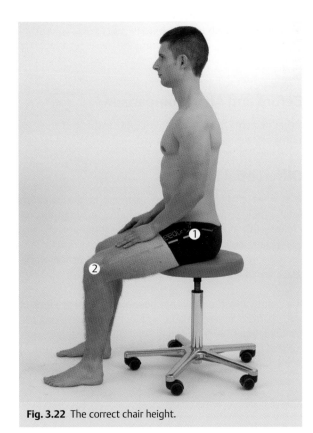

Fig. 3.22 The correct chair height.

How to find the right seat height

If the seat is high enough, sitting up straight becomes easy. If the seat is too high, there is pressure on the back of the thighs or a feeling of slipping forward. The ideal chair height permits easy straightening of the spine without pressure on the back of the thighs or a feeling of slipping forward.

Troubleshooting

The seat of a nonadjustable chair can be raised with cushions. If there is no cushion handy, the patient can lower her knees by placing her feet under the chair. However, this should only be a short-term solution, since this leg position provides less stability, promotes tight hamstrings, and raises the pressure on the patellofemoral joint.

Before and After Comparison

For what percentage of the time seated are the hips higher than the knees?

Differential Diagnosis

If raising the level of the seat causes back pain, it may be because the table height was not raised accordingly, so that the patient now has to compensate by slouching.

On the other hand, if there is a stenosis in the lumbar spine, the improved straightening of the spine resulting from the raised seat level can lead to more back and leg symptoms, since straightening the spine reduces the lumen of the spinal canal. In this case, it is useful to lower the seat height until the symptoms disappear, even if the hips are then no longer higher than the knees.

Biomechanics

A seat is too high if the full weight of the feet cannot be placed on the floor. In this position, the front edge of the seat presses into the posterior thigh, which is not only uncomfortable, but also impedes venous return from the legs. If the patient tries to avoid this pressure by sliding to the forward edge, she will have the feeling of slipping forward. If she tries to reduce the pressure by raising her heels, she will have to hold part of the weight of her legs with the iliopsoas muscles. If this tension becomes habitual, dysfunction of the hip joints, groin, lumbar spine, and respiration may result.

If the seat is too low, the angle of hip flexion is so great that it causes pressure anterior to the axis of hip flexion and, posterior to this, elastic tension in the hip extensors. Both forces counteract an erect pelvic posture and thus a neutral spinal curvature (p. 12). The angle of hip flexion at which insufficient flexibility of the hip extensors becomes an impediment varies considerably from one individual to the next and can be improved by exercising buttock muscle flexibility (p. 96). Therefore, it makes little sense to recommend a specific hip flexion angle as patients would in any case have a hard time measuring this on themselves.

3.8 Distance between the Knees and between the Feet while Seated

Test

Are your feet and your knees positioned apart by about the length of your forearm (**Fig. 3.23**)?

Exercise

Make sure that when you are seated your feet and your knees are positioned apart by about the length of your forearm.

Troubleshooting

If hip abduction mobility is insufficient to position the feet and knees further apart than the hips, see whether this can be improved by exercising inner thigh flexibility (p. 106).

Before and After Comparison

For what percentage of the time seated are the feet and knees apart by about the length of a forearm?

Differential Diagnosis

An excessive distance between the knees and between the feet is never seen in practice, while an insufficient distance is common. There can be many reasons for this. Usually, patients with an insufficient distance are complying with social conventions. For instance, they cross their legs in order to appear elegant or demure. This leg position increases tension in the hip adductors. In time, crossing one's legs, even outside the social context, becomes a habit and can eventually lead to contractures. A positive inner thigh flexibility test indicates contractures and habitual tension of the adductors (p. 106). In this case, the pelvic floor muscles or the iliopsoas muscle are often also tensed. A splinting reflex of these muscles as a result of bladder, kidney, gallbladder, liver, intestinal, or stomach inflammation can also be the primary cause of an insufficient distance between the knees and between the feet, or the cause of diffuse back pain. For this reason, if the distance between the knees or between the feet is too small and there is diffuse back pain, it is advisable to be alert for the following signs of inflammation:

- Bladder: burning during urination and a frequent urge to urinate
- Kidney: elicitation of pain by light percussion with the fist in the kidney region
- Liver: yellow discoloration of the skin and sclera
- Gallbladder: colicky pains after eating fatty foods
- Intestine: bloating, constipation, diarrhea, abdominal pain, or relief after bowel movement
- Stomach: heartburn, black stools, upper abdominal pain increasing with hunger, stress, or the consumption of coffee, alcohol, or cigarettes

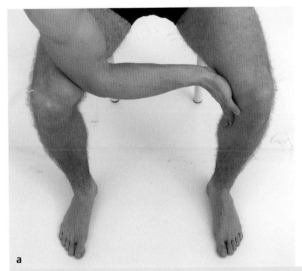 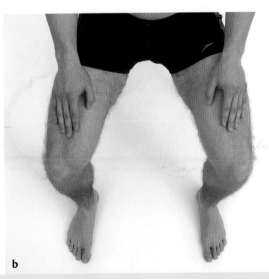

a   b

Fig. 3.23 The length of a forearm (**a**) is the right distance between both the knees and the feet (**b**).

Biomechanics

Like the correct seat height, a wider distance between the knees opens the way for an anterior pelvic tilt and thus for a neutral spinal curvature. Have your patient try out how much harder an erect posture is if she presses her knees together or crosses her legs.

3.9 Symmetrical Weight Distribution when Sitting

Test

Is your weight evenly distributed between both buttocks (**Fig. 3.24 b**), and is the weight of both legs resting completely on the floor (**Fig. 3.25 b**)?

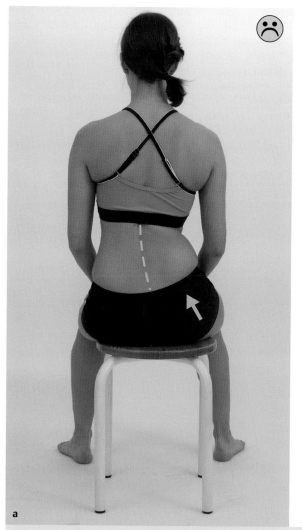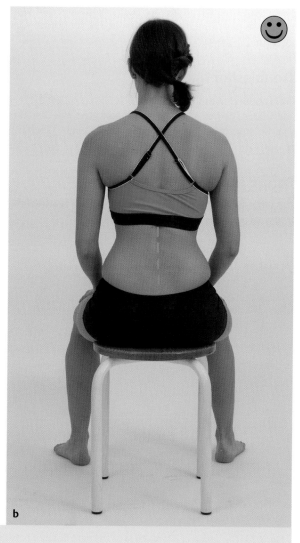

Fig. 3.24 Uneven (**a**) and even (**b**) loading of the buttocks.

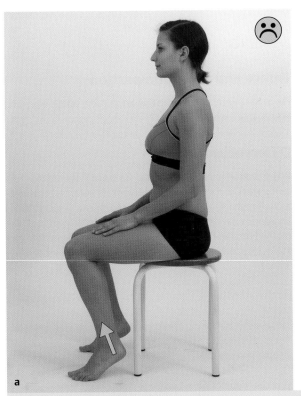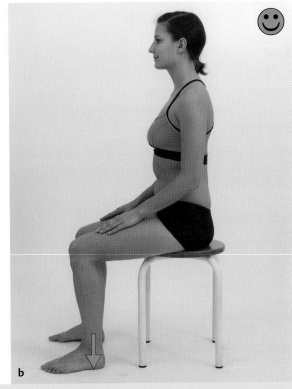

Fig. 3.25 Tensed (**a**) and relaxed (**b**) leg positions.

Exercise

Be sure that your weight is evenly distributed between both buttocks when you are seated (**Fig. 3.24 b**), and that the weight of both legs is resting completely on the floor (**Fig. 3.25 b**).

▶ **Alternative exercise.** If you are not sure whether your weight is evenly distributed, it is usually helpful to shift your weight from side to side and alternately load the left and right buttock a few times, before settling for the middle position in which the pressure is evenly divided between both buttocks.

Troubleshooting

In cases of scoliosis, the spine can feel unbalanced when the weight is evenly distributed over both buttocks. If this feeling persists, a slight imbalance between the buttocks may be required for the sake of keeping the spine balanced.

Before and After Comparison

For what percentage of the time seated is the weight evenly distributed between both buttocks and the weight of both legs fully resting on the floor?

Differential Diagnosis

The patient may perceive an imbalance due to a changed perception or to an actual shift in balance. For instance, if the sciatic nerve lateral to the ischial tuberosity is inflamed, the increased sensitivity may cause the pressure on this side to be perceived as being more intense than it really is. When the patient is sitting, the therapist can feel whether the weight distribution is really unequal, if he places his hand under the patient's ischial tuberosities. Typical causes of uneven weight distribution that should be ruled out are scoliosis, asymmetrical postural habits at work or in the patient's leisure time, dysfunction of the iliosacral joints, an asymmetrical muscle mass in the buttock muscles, or a shift in weight in order to avoid pain.

Biomechanics

An even weight distribution while seated serves to prevent scoliotic deformation, tense spinal muscles, and iliosacral instability. Fully resting the weight of the feet on the floor relaxes the iliopsoas muscle. This removes stress from the hip joints and the lumbar spine and facilitates abdominal breathing (p. 47).

3.10 Stance Width

Test

Are your feet separated by about the width of a shoe (**Fig. 3.26**)?

Exercise

When standing, plant your feet far enough apart so that a third shoe could fit between the two shoes you are wearing (**Fig. 3.26**).

Troubleshooting

In balance disorders caused by a deficient sense of balance or the effect of outside forces (such as turbulent seas), a wider stance could be necessary in order to maintain balance. If the patient has a balance disorder, an attempt should be made to restore a normal stance width by means of balance training.

For patients with an extraordinarily wide pelvis, more than a single shoe width between the feet may be necessary. The therapist should then instruct the patient to leave a space of a "shoe width plus." The instruction to leave a "hip-wide" space between their feet is not helpful for most patients because it is usually not clear which part of the hips is meant or how this distance should be applied to the feet.

Before and After Comparison

For what percentage of the day are the feet about one shoe width apart when standing?

Differential Diagnosis

If the stance is too narrow, for instance with the feet directly next to each other, keeping one's balance is more of a challenge. As a result, the hip and pelvic floor muscles become tense because they must constantly stay at the ready. For this reason, if the hip and pelvic floor muscles are overly tense, a possible cause is an insufficiently wide stance.

On the other hand, a stance that is too wide overloads the arches and the first metatarsophalangeal joints and can cause various foot deformities. For this reason, if deformities of this kind are present, the width of the stance should also be investigated.

You can determine whether a stance that is too wide is compensating for a balance deficit by having the patient correct the width of her stance. If it is now visibly or subjectively harder for her to keep her balance, this is a sign of a balance deficit. In this case, the cause of the balance deficit should be identified and treated.

Biomechanics

With a space of a shoe's width between the feet, the distance between the feet corresponds approximately to the distance between the hip joints, making the axes of the legs parallel to each other. This parallel position has the advantage that the pelvis remains level even if the weight is shifted to one side. In addition, the correct stance width relieves pressure on the hip and foot joints, and facilitates stable dynamic standing.

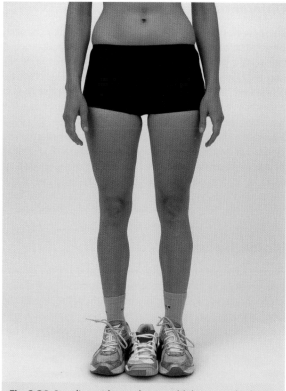

Fig. 3.26 Standing with one shoe's width between the feet.

3.11 Symmetrical Weight Distribution when Standing

Test

How is your weight distributed when you are standing? Do you stand with the same amount of weight on each foot? And do you load the weight evenly on your heels and the balls of your feet?

Exercise

During everyday activities, try to stand with the same amount of weight on each foot (compare **Figs. 3.27**, **3.28**, **3.29**), and on your heels and the balls of your feet (compare **Fig. 3.30 a–c**). This posture should not be rigidly maintained but should be the midpoint of a dynamic posture from which you constantly and regularly shift your weight in all directions. For instance, you can shift your weight alternately from front to back (**Fig. 3.30 a–c**) or from side to side (**Figs. 3.27**, **3.28**, **3.29**). Make sure, however, that you do not habitually keep your weight shifted in the same direction away from the middle (left, right, front, or back). You can find out whether or not this is the case with the following awareness exercises.

Awareness exercise: Left–right weight distribution

You can feel whether or not your weight is shifted to one side by checking the tension in your hip muscles. To do this, place your hands on your hips just below the iliac crest on each side (**Fig. 3.28**). Now with your spine erect, shift your weight to the left by moving your shoulders and pelvis equally far to the left, keeping your knees extended (**Fig. 3.29**). If you shift your weight to the left in this way, you will feel with your left hand that the left hip muscles become tense (**Fig. 3.29**, ①). Conversely, if you shift your weight to the right, you will feel that the muscles of the right hip become tense (**Fig. 3.27**, ②). Now find the middle position, in which both sides feel relatively relaxed (**Fig. 3.28**). In this middle position, your weight is evenly distributed between left and right. This should be the midpoint of your dynamic posture. With a little practice, you will learn to feel, without using your hands, the tension in your hip muscles when you shift your weight to one side or the other.

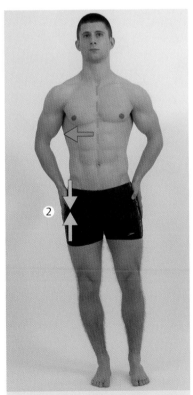

Fig. 3.27 If the weight is shifted to the right, the right hip muscles are tense.

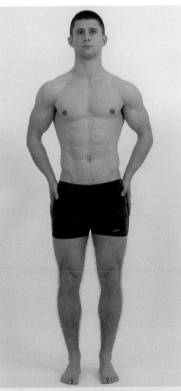

Fig. 3.28 If the weight is distributed symmetrically, the hip muscles are relaxed.

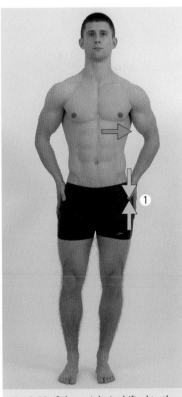

Fig. 3.29 If the weight is shifted to the left, the left hip muscles are tense.

Awareness exercise: Front–back weight distribution

You can *feel* whether your weight is evenly distributed between your heels and the balls of your feet (**Fig. 3.30 b**) through the muscle tension in your lower leg. If your weight is situated too far to the back, toward your heels, the muscles in your shins and the back of your feet are tense (**Fig. 3.30 c**). If you have shifted your weight too far forward toward the balls of your feet, your calf muscles will be tense (**Fig. 3.30 a**).

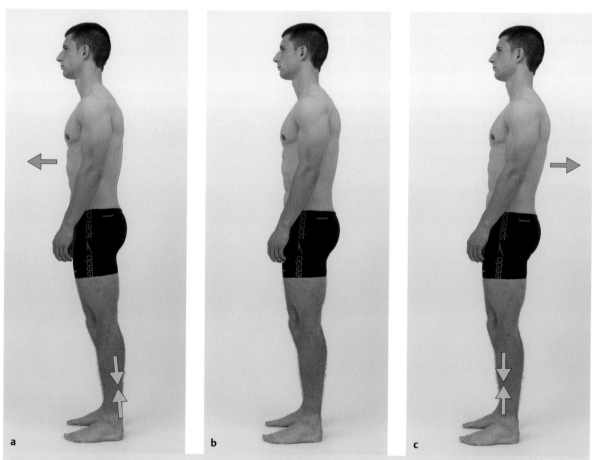

a   b   c

Fig. 3.30 If the weight is shifted forward, away from the midpoint, the calf muscles will become tense (**a**). When the patient stands with his weight evenly distributed, his calf and shin muscles will be relaxed (**b**). If the patient's weight is shifted backward, away from this midpoint, the shin muscles will become tense (**c**).

► **Alternative exercise.** If you have trouble feeling your shin muscles tensing up as soon as your weight is shifted off center backward onto your heels, you can also *see* the tension of your shin muscles if you stand barefoot facing a mirror: the very moment you shift your weight too far backward, a tendon at the very bottom of the shin will pop out and become clearly visible. Correct this by shifting your weight forward until the tendon visibly relaxes.

Troubleshooting

Uneven weight distribution between the left and right foot may be part of the body's attempt to compensate for a leg length discrepancy and keep the pelvis level.

Check for a leg length discrepancy with a measuring device (**Fig. 3.31**). If you find a leg length discrepancy, correct it, either partly or completely depending on where the response of the body's function and structure is most beneficial. The correction usually facilitates an equal weight distribution.

Before and After Comparison

For what percentage of the day is the weight evenly distributed over both feet?

Differential Diagnosis

A leg length discrepancy is not easy to determine visually. In a study of 150 patients, the visual and X-ray results were compared. The visual estimate missed 43% of leg length discrepancy in the clinically relevant range of 6 to 10 mm (Kerr et al 1943).

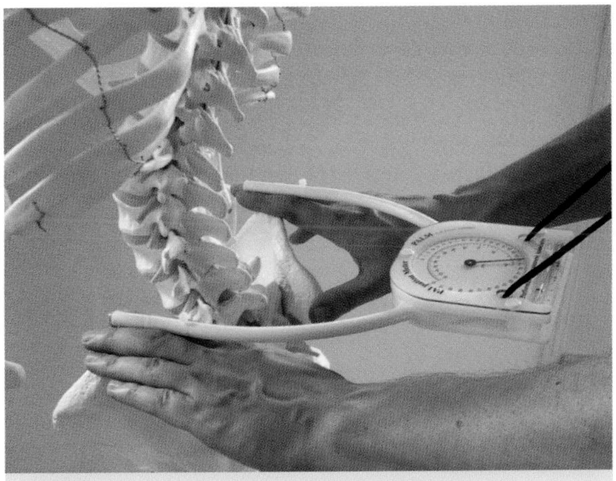

A more exact agreement with the X-ray image is possible using a PALM (Palpation Meter) (Petrone et al 2003). The PALM (**Fig. 3.31**) is a measuring device that provides objective measurement data while it follows the fingers of a therapist as he palpates the bony landmarks.

If the therapist places his fingers with the PALM on the iliac crest (**Fig. 3.31**) while the patient shifts her weight to the left and to the right, the effect of this weight shift on pelvic obliquity can be measured.

The extent to which a leg length discrepancy is structural or functional can be determined with the following mobility exercises: rotational mobility (p. 90), buttock muscle flexibility (p. 96), posterior thigh flexibility (p. 101), inner thigh flexibility (p. 106), hip extension mobility (p. 109), and anterior thigh flexibility (p. 113). The extent to which a leg length discrepancy is reduced by these exercises equals the extent to which the discrepancy is functional.

► **Two-scale test.** Have your patient stand on two identical scales (**Fig. 3.32**) without looking at the display and let her find the muscular balance of her hip abductors by means of palpation (see **Fig. 3.28**). Once your patient tells you she has found her muscular balance, check the scales. If the scales confirm that the weight is evenly distributed between the left and right feet in this position, the palaption method is a valid one for your patient.

Fig. 3.31 Measurement of pelvic tilt using the PALM.

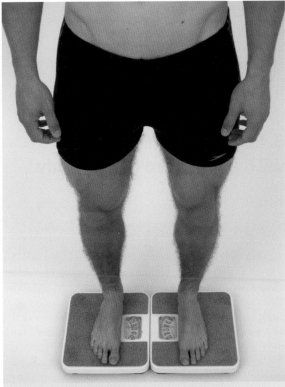
Fig. 3.32 The two-scale test.

If this is not the case, you should take over the palpation of muscular equilibrium (see **Fig. 3.28**). If both scales now show the same weight, the patient was clearly not yet able to find his muscular equilibrium on his own and should continue to practice this with you.

If the scales still show unequal weights even when you determine that the hip abductors are in equilibrium, the muscles are probably compensating for some other asymmetry. If this is impossible to find and correct, it is usually more advantageous to keep the spine in muscular equilibrium (see **Fig. 3.28**) rather than insisting on having an equal pressure exerted by both feet. But it should always be determined in each individual case whether the equilibrium of the hip muscles or an equal pressure distribution between the feet serves to provide the greatest improvements in the patient's function and symptoms.

Biomechanics

Provided that the leg length is even, standing with an equal weight distribution promotes the muscular equilibrium of the legs and torso, the stability of the pelvic joints, and a neutral spinal position in the frontal plane.

Comparing the weight distribution between the left and right feet on the basis of the sense of pressure on both heels is less exact than the palpation of muscular equilibrium described above (see **Fig. 3.28**). This is because the sense of touch in the fingers is significantly more exact than the sense of pressure in the heels. In addition, the sense of pressure in the heels can change if an unequal weight distribution has persisted for a long time. Finally, a change in heel pressure can only be felt on a hard surface. Therefore, this method of checking weight distribution is not suitable for people wearing shoes with soft soles.

3.12 Standing Posture with a Balanced Upper Body

Test

Is your upper body balanced when you are standing?

In order to find the answer to this question, first feel the tension in your abdominal muscles by pressing the fingers of your left hand slightly into your abdomen, just above your pubic bone (**Fig. 3.33 a–c**, ①). If you do not find your pubic bone, press your fingers into your abdomen at the upper edge of the pubic hair. Place your right hand with the thumb pointing forward on the right iliac crest while the tips of the other fingers lie on the right back extensor muscle (**Fig. 3.33 a–c**, ②) that lies close to your spine as a vertical muscle strand.

Now thrust your pelvis forward until you feel with your fingers how your abdominal muscles tense and push your fingers out of your abdomen, while your back muscles relax (**Fig. 3.33 a**).

Similarly, you can feel with your fingers how your back muscles tense and your abdominal muscles relax when you push your buttocks backward past the middle (**Fig. 3.33 c**).

Now find the middle position between these two, in which the back and abdominal muscles are equally relaxed (**Fig. 3.33 b**). This is the standing posture with a balanced upper body.

In case your habitual posture is characterized by leaning your upper body back while pushing the pelvis forward, the correct balanced posture will at first feel as though the buttocks were protruding too far to the back. If you look at yourself from the side, using two mirrors, or have someone else look at you, you will find that this is not the case. Rather, in the balanced position, you immediately look more upright, more balanced, and slimmer.

Exercise

When you are standing, make sure that your upper body remains close to the vertical.

▶ **Alternative exercise.** Try to see whether you can feel the alternation between abdominal and back muscle tension when you lean backward and forward, even without using your fingers. This trains your body awareness and lets you find the balanced upper body position quickly and inconspicuously during your everyday activities. This awareness exercise will soon teach you that the tension also changes in many other muscles when you lean forward or backward.

Troubleshooting

If your patient is not able to feel the alternation of muscle tension between the anterior and posterior muscle chain, you should check whether she has in fact placed her fingers on the erector spinae and rectus abdominis muscles. In very overweight patients, the superior end of the rectus abdominis directly under the xiphoid process may be felt more easily than its inferior end.

> ### Pushing instead of tipping
>
> Alternation of muscle tension is only palpable if the patient does not tilt her pelvis while searching for the balanced upper body position but pushes it in relaxed fashion past the middle position, forward and backward.

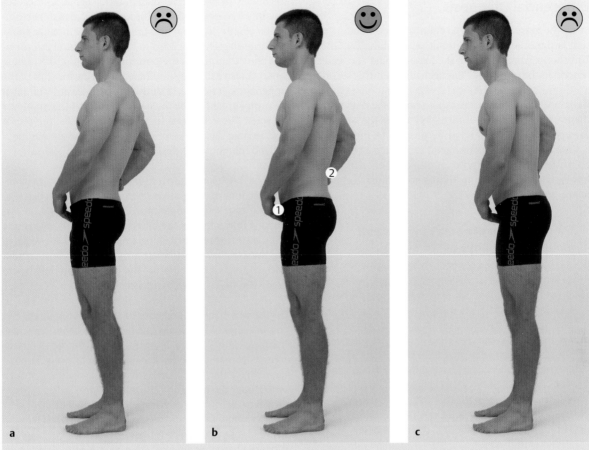

Fig. 3.33 Standing position with the pelvis too far forward (**a**), balanced (**b**), and too far backward (**c**).

If, shortly after posture correction, your patient immediately returns to a posture with an anterior pelvic shift, it may be that she is compensating for an extension deficit in the thoracic spine. In the case of a deficit in thoracic spine extension, bringing the upper body and pelvis into balanced alignment will cause the line of sight to tilt downward. In order to raise the line of sight again, either the pelvis will have to be shifted forward and/or the cervical spine will have to be hyperextended. For this reason, thoracic extension mobility (p. 73) should also always be tested in patients who stand with an anterior pelvic shift. If the test is positive, restoring full thoracic extension mobility (p. 73) is essential for enabling a patient to look straight ahead with a balanced and neutral posture.

If your patient compensates for an extension deficit in the thoracic spine by shifting her pelvis forward, she needs to be instructed to both realign her pelvis and straighten her thoracic spine. This corrected posture with a balanced upper body will seem markedly overcorrected to her. The patient will only feel motivated to maintain this posture in her everyday life if she can be shown, with two mirrors, that the corrected posture does not look as funny as it feels but actually looks better and instantly slims her belly down.

Before and After Comparison

For what percentage of the day is the upper body close to the vertical while standing?

Differential Diagnosis

By far the most frequent type of unbalanced standing posture is the one with an anterior pelvic shift (**Fig. 3.33 a**). This causes compression of the lumbar spine and leads to tension in the groin (see "Biomechanics" for this section).

If compression of the lumbar spine causes local symptoms, these usually improve immediately when the posture is corrected. On the other hand, because nerve regeneration is slow, it can only be determined some time after posture correction whether the anterior displacement of the pelvis has caused paresthesia in the lateral femoral cutaneous nerve (see text box below).

Paresthesia in the area of the lateral femoral cutaneous nerve

It can be decided on the basis of location whether a paresthesia of the lateral femoral cutaneous nerve is being caused peripherally or in the region of the nerve roots at L1 and L2. If the damage is peripheral, the lateral cutaneous femoral nerve is usually compressed in the muscular lacuna. This causes a wide area of paresthesia on the lateral thigh. On the other hand, a herniated disk usually compresses only one of the two nerve roots (L1 or L2) of the lateral cutaneous femoral nerve. The resulting paresthesia then follows the narrower band of the L1 or L2 dermatome. Other indications of nerve compression in the area of the nerve root are easing of the parasthesia in the lateral thigh with traction of the lumbar spine, and an increase in parasthesia with ipsilateral lateral flexion of the lumbar spine.

Biomechanics

With equal relaxation of the anterior and posterior muscle chains, balanced upper body posture relieves the pressure on the disks and prevents rapid tiring and tension of the trunk and hip muscles. In contrast, since the torque required to equilibrate the trunk musculature in the balanced upper body position is approaching zero, an upright posture here becomes effortless. This makes the balanced upper body an ideal midpoint of a dynamic posture. In addition, hyperextension of the knees while standing is automatically resolved when the upper body is balanced.

In contrast, a posture with an anterior pelvic shift causes not only hyperextension of the knees, but also unnecessary tension in the groin and pressure in the lumbar spine. Shifting the pelvis forward increases the lumbar lordosis and thus compresses the posterior portion of the lumbar spine. It also causes a simultaneous backward shift of the upper body in relation to the hip. This backward shift must be compensated for by increased tension of the hip flexor muscles. These muscles include the iliopsoas, the tensor fasciae latae, and the anterior portions of the gluteus medius and minimus muscles.

Increased tension in the tensor fasciae latae and the anterior portions of the gluteus medius and minimus can lead to persistent local symptoms in these muscles and the fascia lata. Correction of the anterior pelvic shift is then the only way to produce lasting improvement. However, if the muscles have been tense for years, any improvement with consistent correction of the posture will only be felt gradually, from month to month.

On the one hand, hypertonus of the iliopsoas intensifies compression of the lumbar spine. On the other hand, the hardness and volume increase of the tensed iliopsoas muscle can impinge on the lateral cutaneous femoral nerve in the narrow space of the muscular lacuna, through which both the nerve and the muscle run.

Another vulnerable site for the lateral cutaneous femoral nerve is at its emergence from the muscular lacuna, where it bends sharply downward. This bend is intensified by an anterior pelvic shift and stresses the nerve at this point as well. If the stress persists long enough, the typical consequence is a feeling of numbness in the lateral thigh (see "Differential Diagnosis" for this section).

Flexing the hip relieves the strain on the lateral cutaneous femoral nerve. The relief is due to the fact that the kink at the emergence from the muscular lacuna is diminished with hip flexion. In addition, the iliopsoas also relaxes when the hip is flexed, thus leaving more space for the nerve within the muscular lacuna.

Correction of an anterior pelvic shift while standing removes stress from the lateral cutaneous femoral nerve and gives it a chance to recover, but since nerves recover very slowly, this can take weeks or months if the numbness has existed for a long time.

4 Relaxation

Relaxing cramped muscles removes stress from the underlying joints, nerves, lymph vessels, and blood vessels. Moreover, relaxing the muscles decreases the resistance to blood flow within the muscles, which also improves their perfusion.

Contracting and relaxing is not a local event of a single muscle; it proceeds like the toppling of a line of dominos, as a process chain that branches along various muscles throughout the body. Because of this branching, it is, with a little training, possible to feel how relaxing the functional muscle chain tongue–lower jaw–lower lip–shoulders–abdomen simultaneously relaxes other muscles as well including the entire back musculature.

4.1 Relaxed Tongue

Test

Is your tongue relaxed and lying at a little distance from your front teeth, in the wide part of your mouth (**Fig. 4.1**)?

Exercise

Make sure that your tongue is lying so relaxed within your mouth that the tip of your tongue is in the wide part of your mouth and at a little distance from your front teeth when it is not being used for other activities such as eating, drinking, or speaking.

If your jaw feels relaxed, you have found the right resting position for your tongue. If your tongue feels too long in the relaxed position, you can restore a sense of proper length by dropping your lower jaw a little more (p. 41).

▶ **Alternative exercises.** The definition of the tongue's position at a little distance from the front teeth is purposely inexact, in order to leave you leeway to find your own resting position intuitively. An objective of this resting position is relaxation of the jaw muscles. If you do not reach this by means of an intuitively selected tongue position, place the front of your tongue in the natural resting position against the palate at a little distance from the incisors of the upper jaw. If you are not sure how large this distance should be, you should select the distance at which your jaw muscles feel the most relaxed. An alternative description that also helps to find the natural tongue position with relaxed jaw muscles is described in the following box.

> #### How to find the right resting position for your tongue
>
> Let the anterior third of your tongue glide upward until it lightly touches your palate about a centimeter behind your front teeth (**Fig. 4.1**), while letting the posterior two-thirds of your tongue go slack like a hammock. If this is the tongue position with which you pronounce the letter "L" you can also think of this as the "L-position."
>
> The resting position of the tongue described here only applies to sitting and standing. When you are lying on your back, relax completely, and simply let your whole tongue and lower jaw slide back with gravity.

Troubleshooting

If your patient cannot arrive at the feeling of a relaxed jaw with either the exercise or the alternative exercise, she may succeed if, at the same time, she pays attention to the following:
- Neutral spinal curvature (p. 12)
- Relaxed lower jaw (p. 41)
- Relaxed lower lip (p. 43)
- Abdominal breathing (p. 47)

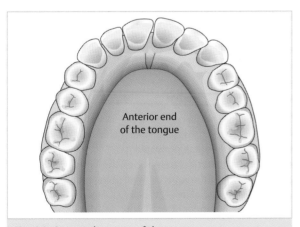

Anterior end of the tongue

Fig. 4.1 Correct placement of the tongue.

With mouth breathing, it is not possible to have the tongue contact the palate as described in the alternative exercise. If you observe that your patient often breathes with an open mouth, you should ask her whether she gets enough air through her nose with her mouth closed. If not, you may suggest that nose breathing is maintained consistently for 5 minutes, which will usually open the nasal pathways.

Before and After Comparison

For what percentage of the time is the tongue in a relaxed position without contact with the front teeth?

Differential Diagnosis

Most patients are not conscious of their tongue position. For this reason, when their medical history is taken, they will not be able to say whether their tongue touches the incisors only momentarily or habitually. The therapist, however, can determine this by inspecting the tongue.

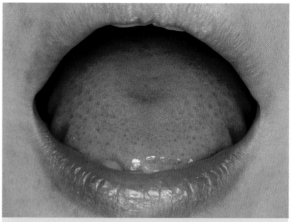

Fig. 4.2 Imprints of the teeth at the edge of the tongue.

Tongue findings

If contact with the incisors is habitual, there are imprints of the teeth along the edge of the tongue (**Fig. 4.2**). The exact location of the imprints indicate whether the patient is in the habit of pressing her tongue forward, to one side, or between the side teeth. The imprints disappear at the slightest tensing of the tongue. Thus, they are only visible as long as the tongue is completely relaxed and lying on the floor of the mouth (**Fig. 4.2**). To see the imprints, the therapist should therefore ask the patient to open her mouth without mentioning the tongue. If the tongue is mentioned, the patient will inevitably extend her tongue or tense it some other way.

Biomechanics

The physiological resting position of the tongue at the palate described under "Alternative Exercises" for this section is a prerequisite for normal development of the upper jaw. If this tongue contact is missing during growth, the upper jaw does not take on a sufficiently wide shape. As a result, there is not enough space for free nose breathing and normal alignment of the upper teeth.

After the termination of growth, tongue placement at the upper jaw also has advantages. For one thing, most people find that this gives them a more relaxed jaw position. In addition, this tongue position serves as an airtight partition between the front and back of the oral cavity. This protects the teeth, which are bathed in saliva in the front of the oral cavity, from being dried out by the respiratory airstream in the back of the oral cavity. This is beneficial because the saliva contains minerals, antibodies, and acid-balancing buffers that prevent caries and gum inflammation.

The most frequent parafunction of the tongue is to push forward against the teeth. This anterior pressure of the tongue displaces the teeth and leads to a gap between the tooth and the gum, which exposes the sensitive neck of the tooth to acids and cold, serves as a habitat for bacteria.

Parafunction

In dentistry, parafunction is a term for nonfunctional activities of the chewing muscles or the tongue. This includes, among other things, grinding and gritting the teeth or the above-mentioned pressing of the tongue against the front teeth.

Moreover, the tongue cannot exert an anterior pressure against the incisors without co-contraction of the lateral pterygoid muscle to counteract the posterior reaction force of the incisors.

Lateral pterygoid muscle

With time, habitual tension of the lateral pterygoid muscle promotes a number of symptoms and dysfunctions:

- A painful irritation of the muscle itself
- Tinnitus
- A feeling of pressure in the ear
- Tension between the sphenoid bone and its adjacent skull bones via the tension at origin of the pterygoid
- Osteophytes at the mandibular head via the pull of the inferior head of the pterygoid
- Antero-medial displacement of the interarticular disk via the pull of the superior head of the pterygoid
- Temporomandibular joint pain, clicking, popping, and locking as a result of the anterior disk displacement

4.2 Relaxed Lower Jaw

Test

Seated or standing: Is your lower jaw hanging loosely with gravity so that your cheeks feel relaxed and there is a large distance between your upper and lower teeth (compare **Figs. 4.3** and **4.4**)?

Lying on your back: Can gravity make your relaxed lower jaw slide straight back behind the upper jaw (compare **Figs. 4.5** and **4.6**)?

Exercise

In everyday life, let your lower jaw hang loose while your lips remain lightly touching (**Figs. 4.4** and **4.6**).

Troubleshooting

If your patient is having trouble letting her lower jaw fall loosely, it is often easier if she pays attention to the following at the same time:
- Neutral spinal curvature (p. 12)
- Relaxed lower lip (p. 43)
- Relaxed tongue (p. 39)
- Abdominal breathing (p. 47)
- Relaxed shoulders (p. 45)

Using manual intraoral myofascial release techniques on the muscles of mastication can also help by giving the patient a sense of what a relaxed jaw feels like.

Before and After Comparison

For what percentage of the time is the lower jaw relaxed in everyday life?

Differential Diagnosis

Parafunctional hypertonia of the jaw muscles may be reflex induced, compensatory, part of a tense muscle chain, or caused by stress.

Reflex hypertonia can be caused by pain or a hematoma. If it is caused by pain, a distinction must be made between the muscles and the teeth as source of the pain. If the jaw muscles are only painful because of a parafunction, the tension can be resolved with conscious relaxation exercises (pp. 39–49) and manual myofascial release techniques.

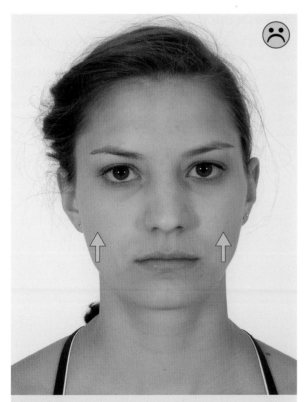

Fig. 4.3 Tense jaw muscles with the teeth too close together.

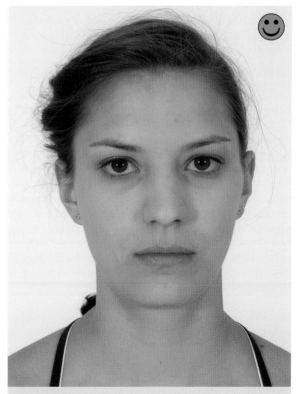

Fig. 4.4 Relaxed jaw muscles where the teeth are far apart.

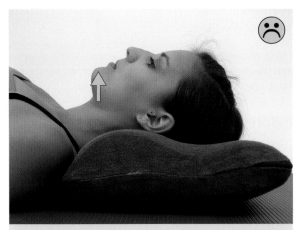

Fig. 4.5 When you slide your lower jaw forward, your jaw muscles are distinctly tenser ...

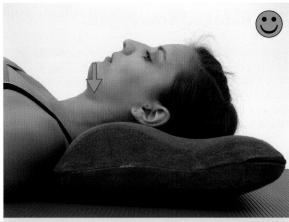

Fig. 4.6 ... than if you let your relaxed lower jaw slide backward with gravity.

Hypodermic hematoma

If you cannot open your mouth naturally after injection of a local anesthetic by the dentist, but there is no sign of a mandibular joint blockade, it is necessary to determine whether a blood vessel has been hit, causing a hematoma in the affected muscle, usually the masseter. If there is in fact a hematoma, the usual physiotherapeutic treatments are ineffectual. If the hematoma is not infected, the problem will resolve itself spontaneously by gradual, natural absorption of the hematoma over the course of about 6 weeks. An infected hematoma only disappears with the administration of antibiotics.

If the reflex tension of the jaw muscles is caused by a painful defect of the teeth or gums, it can only be corrected by dental treatment to eliminate the pain. This tooth pain can only be relieved slightly, and for a maximum of 10 minutes, by conscious relaxation or a manual reduction of tension in the jaw muscles. On the other hand, if the teeth and gums are healthy and habitual tensing of the jaw muscles is the only cause of the tooth pain, this pain is immediately significantly reduced for several hours by a manual reduction of tension in the jaw muscles. If a patient becomes accustomed to a relaxed resting mouth position, this kind of tooth pain will disappear permanently, even without further treatment.

Compensatory tension of the jaw muscles in response to slouching can be resolved to the extent that neutral spinal curvature (p. 12) is adopted. The biomechanical connections between posture and jaw muscle tone are described in the section on biomechanics.

If the tense muscles are part of a tension chain, they relax more easily if other muscles in the chain are also relaxed (pp. 26 and 39–49).

Stress-based tension is naturally intensified or decreased with shifting stress levels. For instance, if the principal stress factor is work, the medical history shows that the tension is greater on work days than on days off.

Biomechanics

The lower teeth should only touch the upper teeth during swallowing and chewing. Frequent contact at other times overloads the muscles of mandibular elevation (masseter, medial pterygoid, and temporal muscle), the mandibular joints, and the ears. By the same token, the prognosis is good for symptoms in these areas if a patient becomes re-accustomed to letting her lower jaw hang loose.

Lasting relaxation

Lasting relaxation of hypertonic jaw muscles is only possible if the excessive tone is not reflex induced, compensatory, or part of a tension chain that is not caused by the jaw muscles.

Relation between posture and chewing muscle tone

The most frequent cause of compensatory tightening of the muscles of mastication is slouching. If the patient wishes to look straight ahead in this posture, she must hyperextend her cervical spine to do so. This results in elastic tension of the supra- and infrahyoidal tissues at the front of the neck. This elastic tension pulls the lower jaw in a dorsal and inferior direction. Some patients give in to this pull by letting the mouth hang open. Most patients, however, resist the pull and keep the jaw set. In this case, they compensate for the inferior pull by increased tension of the muscles of mandibular elevation. Correspondingly, the tone of the muscles that push the lower jaw forward (lateral pterygoid and superficial portion of the masseter) increases as they compensate for the dorsal pull of the hyoid tissue in the slouched posture.

4.3 Relaxed Lower Lip

Test

Does your lower lip hang loosely from your upper lip, so that your upper lip is lightly pulled downward by your lower lip (compare **Figs. 4.7** and **4.8**)?

Exercise

In daily life, let your lower lip hang loosely from your upper lip (**Fig. 4.8**) when it is not needed for functions such as speech or facial expressions. Also be sure that after you smile, you let both your lower lip and the corners of your mouth hang loosely with the pull of gravity. Then at the next opportunity, your smile can unfold again without looking as though it were pasted on your face.

Troubleshooting

If your patient cannot let her lower lip hang loosely at first, she may succeed if, at the same time, she pays attention to the following:
- Neutral spinal curvature (p. 12)
- Relaxed tongue (p. 39)
- Relaxed lower jaw (p. 41)

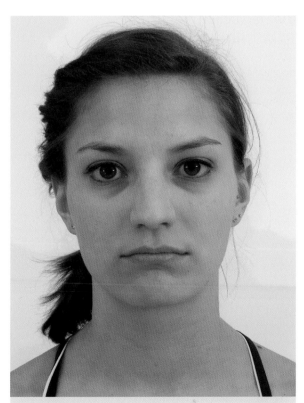

Fig. 4.7 The lower lip is pushed upward by a contraction of the muscle between the lower lip and the tip of the chin.

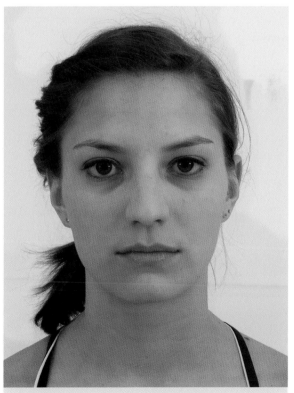

Fig. 4.8 The lower lip hangs loosely from the upper lip.

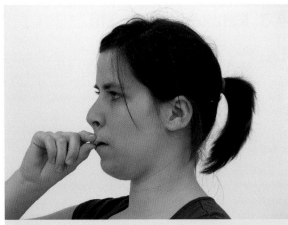

Fig. 4.9 Stretching an upper lip that is too short.

- Relaxed shoulders (p. 45)
- Abdominal breathing (p. 47)

If the patient still does not succeed after these exercises, you should check whether your patient is pushing her lower lip upward in order to compensate for an open bite, an increased horizontal overbite, or a short upper lip (see "Differential Diagnosis" for this section).

An open bite and an increased horizontal overbite can only be corrected with orthodontic treatment. A short upper lip can be stretched (**Fig. 4.9**).

Before and After Comparison

For what percentage of the time does the lower lip hang loosely from the upper lip in everyday life?

Differential Diagnosis

If the distance between lower and upper lip is too great (**Fig. 4.10**), the lips are usually closed by pushing the lower lip up in active compensation (**Fig. 4.11**). An excessively large distance between the lips can be caused by the fact that one or both lips are too short:

- A functionally short lower lip can occur if the anterior cervical fasciae are tense due to slouching (see **Fig. 3.3**) and pull the lower lip down.
- In the case of a short upper lip, the upper lip muscle is so short that the upper incisors are hardly covered or not at all by the upper lip when the mouth is loosely hanging open (**Fig. 4.10**).

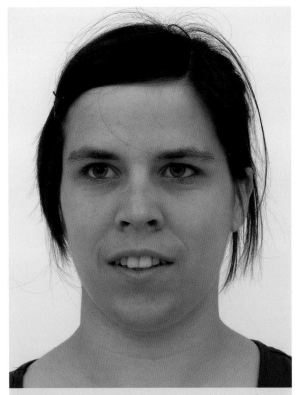

Fig. 4.10 In the relaxed state, a short upper lip covers the upper incisors very little or not at all ...

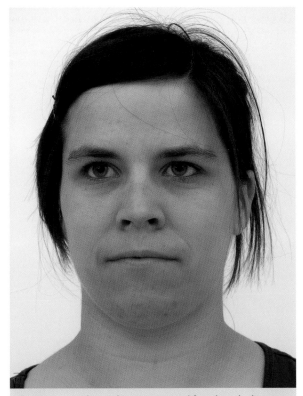

Fig. 4.11 ... and must be compensated for when the lips are closed by tightening of the mentalis muscle.

On the other hand, there can be an excessive distance between the lips, even when they are of normal length, if the upper and lower jaws are too far apart, either vertically or horizontally:

- Normally the incisors of the upper and lower jaw should have a vertical overlap of 2–3 mm when the molars of the upper and lower jaw are in contact. In the case of an anterior open bite, there is no vertical overbite.
- If the horizontal overbite is increased, the horizontal gap between upper and lower incisors is greater than the usual 1 to 2 mm.

Biomechanics

The lower lip is pushed upward by contraction of the mentalis muscle. The lower lip can be pushed up even further if the entire lower jaw is pushed forward along with it, so that these two movements always occur together. The lateral pterygoid muscle is the principal agent in pushing the lower jaw forward. Thus, a lower lip that is pushed upward leads to contraction of the lateral pterygoid muscle with the corresponding result (p. 40, "Biomechanics").

4.4 Relaxed Shoulders

Test

Do your shoulders hang loosely, with gravity, from your upright spine (**Fig. 4.12 a**)?

In the supine position, do your shoulders fall loosely, under their own weight, toward the surface on which you are lying (**Fig. 4.12 b**)?

Exercise

Make sure that your shoulders hang loosely from your erect spine during your everyday activities.

Troubleshooting

If your patient is having trouble letting her shoulders fall loosely, it is often easier if she pays attention to the following at the same time:

- Neutral spinal curvature (p. 12)
- Relaxed lower jaw (p. 41)
- Relaxed lower lip (p. 43)
- Relaxed tongue (p. 39)
- Abdominal breathing (p. 47)
- Letting her elbows hang loosely next to her body

If this is not sufficient, deficits in the following areas should be found and corrected:

- Thoracic extension mobility (p. 73)
- Arm nerve mobility (p. 83)
- Shoulder mobility (p. 78)
- Rotational mobility (p. 90)

If tension increases during certain activities, you should examine whether the ergonomics of the respective activity can be improved. Examples are the particularly damaging habit of clamping the telephone between the shoulder and ear or carrying heavy bags in the hand or over one shoulder. In such cases, a considerable unburdening of the shoulder elevators can be achieved by using a headset while telephoning and a backpack for carrying. The backpack should have a hip belt that is buckled firmly around the pelvis, so that the majority of the weight is not hanging from the shoulders but is carried by the pelvis.

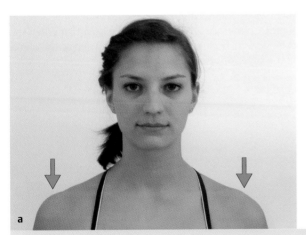
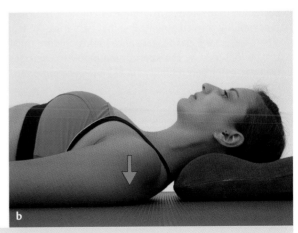

Fig. 4.12 Let your shoulders fall under their own weight.

Before and After Comparison

For what percentage of the day do your patient's shoulders hang loosely from her upright spine?

Differential Diagnosis

Prerequisites for a normal tone in the shoulder elevators are an ergonomic environment (p. 27), abdominal breathing (p. 47), thoracic extension mobility (p. 73), shoulder mobility (p. 78), arm nerve mobility (p. 83), and rotational mobility (p. 90). Deficits in these areas should be found and corrected with the appropriate tests and exercises. If a test objective has been achieved and the shoulders can relax, the cause has been found and eliminated.

- If tension in the neck increases at work, biomechanical and psychological causes need to be destinguished. Biomechanically generated symptoms change when the physical task changes, whereas symptoms with psychological causes are more likely to depend on the workplace culture. For this reason, you should ask to what extent a patient's symptoms depend on the physical task or on the workplace culture.
- A cervical rib is present in only about 1% of the population but can irritate the lower branches of the brachial plexus, leading to a reflex increase in tone of the shoulder elevators. The findings on palpation to rule out a cervical rib are not always conclusive. Only an X-ray provides a certain diagnosis.

Biomechanics

Possible biomechanical causes of parafunctional contraction of the shoulder elevators:

- These muscles may be part of a hypertonic muscle chain. The solution here is to find the key to relaxing this chain by means of the suitable relaxation exercises. Often a relaxed lower jaw (p. 41), relaxed lower lip (p. 43), relaxed tongue (p. 39), and abdominal breathing (p. 47) are keys to relaxation.
- Increased cervical flexion torque due to an anterior displacement of the head: This torque can only be returned to normal by restoring neutral spinal curvature (p. 12). Where necessary, elastic resistance to this posture must first be loosened by the appropriate mobility exercises (thoracic extension mobility [p. 73] and rotational mobility [p. 90]).
- Reflex contraction of the shoulder elevators to protect an irritated brachial plexus. Irritation of the brachial plexus is often the result of increased neural tension and most frequently affects the median nerve. If this is the case, the restriction can be detected and improved with the arm nerve mobility test and exercise (p. 83). If the nerve recovers thanks to the exercise, the tension in the shoulder elevators is automatically relaxed.

- Limited glenohumeral internal rotation that is compensated for by elevation and protraction of the shoulder. A bilateral internal rotation of the glenohumeral joint brings the hands toward the body's midline, as is required for many activities such as using a keyboard. If the internal rotation of the glenohumeral joint is limited, the hands need to be brought toward the body's midline with a compensatory elevation and protraction of the shoulder. It is only with the re-establishment of free shoulder mobility (p. 78) that this compensation becomes unnecessary.
- Intensified torque in the arm because the elbow is not kept loosely next to the trunk. This often happens during computer work, if the mouse or the keyboard is too far away and the lower arm is not supported. The patient can learn to feel the pronounced increase in the tension in her upper trapezius with flexion or abduction of the shoulder joint with the following awareness exercise.

Awareness exercise: Shoulder muscle contraction and relaxation

Sit at a table and place the index and middle fingers of your right hand on your left collarbone. Push these two fingers backward over the collarbone until they reach the muscle that is located there. Feel the difference in tension or relaxation of the muscle in the following positions:

- When your left lower arm lies loosely on the table
- When you raise your left shoulder slightly toward your ear
- When your left arm hangs loosely next to your body
- When you extend your left arm slightly forward
- When you move your left arm slightly sideways, away from your body

If the patient succeeds in becoming accustomed to a posture with relaxed shoulders, the shoulder elevators and the remainder of the muscle chain involved in shoulder elevation can relax. This relieves the load on the muscles themselves and decompresses the cervical spine and the thoracic outlet. Finally, it can often be seen that when the shoulders relax, suboccipital hyperextension at the origin of the superior trapezius also resolves.

4.5 Abdominal Breathing

Test

Does your lower abdomen expand with inhalation (**Fig. 4.13**) while your thorax remains hanging so loosely (from the erect spine) in a relaxed exhalation stage that no movements of your shoulders, thorax, or collar bones are visible in the mirror, when you breathe?

Exercise

Maintain a posture with a neutral spinal curvature (p. 12) and balanced upper body when seated (p. 25) while you pull in your abdomen a little during exhalation and release it again during inhalation, without a rise in your thorax.

▶**Alternative exercises.** Depending on what feels best, the movement of the abdomen during inhalation can be practiced to the front, back, or laterally, or in several of these directions at once. Catching a breath during pauses in speech should be accomplished without a rise in the thorax.

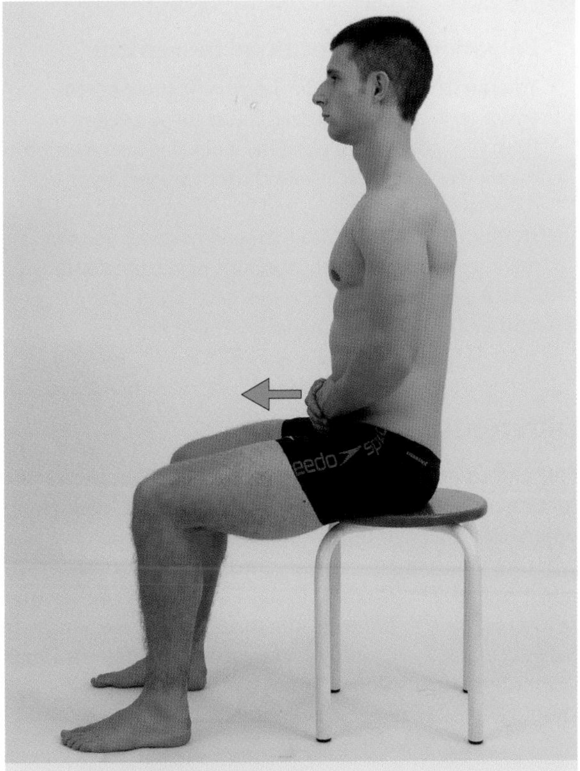

Fig. 4.13 Abdominal breathing.

Breathing during pauses in speech

The patient audibly counts upward in ones—"1, 2, 3 ..." —until she feels a need to inhale. She should do this as described above, with pure abdominal breathing. She does not speak during inhalation. In this way, inhalation becomes a pause in speech. She only continues speaking once the inhalation has been completed.

If the patient is able to do this without raising her thorax during inhalation, she should now switch from counting to describing her plans for the rest of the day, using the same breathing technique. This provides training for the goal of maintaining abdominal breathing while simultaneously carrying on a conversation.

Finally, in the same way, she should speak about the particularly stressful recurrent situations in her life. Usually, the very thought of the stressful situation provokes a relapse into a costosternal breathing pattern. But with time and consistent practice, the patient learns to continue with relatively relaxed breathing even in more stressful situations. This helps her to retain mental concentration and avoid tension-related symptoms.

Troubleshooting

Conversion to pure abdominal breathing rarely occurs spontaneously, but it is feasible with faithful practice and elimination of the following deficits.

- **Slouching**
  If purely abdominal breathing is not possible, the most frequent reason is that the patient abandons a neutral spinal curvature (p. 12) and slouches a bit during exhalation. In this position, the abdominal cavity is compressed so that there is insufficient space for inhalation into the abdomen. Therefore it is very important to start with an exhalation in which the abdomen is pulled in while the spine remains erect. At the start of training, it is helpful to exaggerate the exhalation movement by actively drawing the navel as far as possible toward the spine. To prevent this technique from causing hyperventilation, the navel should remain pulled in at the end of the exhalation movement until the need for the next breath is felt.

- **Hypertonic abdominal muscles**
  If the patient stands or sits with her upper body inclined backward, without leaning against anything, the abdominal muscles must work harder to hold her, which makes abdominal inhalation more difficult. In this case, she should compare to how much easier it feels once she assumes a posture with a balanced upper body (pp. 25 and 36).

- **Pants that are too tight**
  If abdominal breathing in a seated starting position is easier with the pants unbuttoned, the pants are too tight. To eliminate symptoms caused by costosternal inhalation, the patient must buy pants that are so loose that abdominal inhalation is equally easy with the pants open or closed. This should be checked in the fitting room of the store. If the patient intends to lose weight, she should still buy at least one pair of loose pants, since diet plans are usually put into effect slowly, only for a short while, or not at all.

- **Vanity**
  Many people keep their abdominal muscles tensed or confine their bellies in pants that are too tight, in the belief that they will look slimmer that way. Explain to your patient that this is the wrong idea. Relaxed abdominal breathing massages, loosens, and perfuses all the abdominal organs, including the intestines. If there is no abdominal breathing, the intestine becomes prone to constipation and bloating, both of which may cause the abdomen to expand markedly. Therefore, it is important to let the abdomen breathe and live. If the abdomen feels unpleasantly fat and bloated when it is released during breathing in, it should not be confined by means of muscle tension. The better solution is a diet that makes the abdomen feel at ease and healthy.

- **Difficulty breathing**
  When a habitual costosternal breathing pattern is eliminated, most patients have the feeling, at first, that they are not getting enough air. This feeling of insufficiency disappears immediately if attention is shifted from the absence of the old breathing movement to the new abdominal breathing. In fact, conversion to abdominal breathing induces a deeper, slower kind of breathing that consumes less energy and increases performance capability (Mead and Loring 1982, Jones et al 2003, Vickery 2007).

- **Chain of tension**
  If the orofacial musculature is tense, abdominal breathing is more difficult. Have your patient experience how much easier abdominal breathing is with a relaxed lower jaw (p. 41), tongue (p. 39), and lower lip (p. 43) than when the teeth are touching, the tongue is pressing forward against the teeth, and the lower lip is pushing the upper lip upward.

Before and After Comparison

For what percentage of the time is the patient practicing abdominal breathing (as described above)?

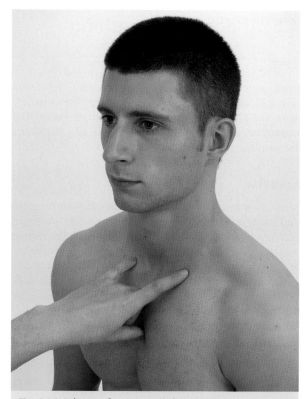

Fig. 4.14 Palpation for costosternal movement.

Palpation for costosternal movement

You can determine the short-term effect of your instruction in abdominal breathing as follows. Sit across from your patient and place the index finger of your left hand on his left clavicle with the little finger of your left hand on his right clavicle, and your right thumb on his sternum (**Fig. 4.14**). With this hand position, you can feel precisely whether the thorax is rising on inhalation. Compare how much of this movement you can feel before and after the abdominal breathing exercise.

Differential Diagnosis

Full extension of the thoracic spine is an important requirement for relaxed abdominal breathing. Therefore, when costosternal breathing is present, always check whether your patient can pass the thoracic extension mobility test (p. 73). Thoracic extension is often irreversibly restricted by compression fractures or diseases such as Scheuermann syndrome or ankylosing spondylitis. Pure diaphragmatic inhalation is impossible in such cases and should therefore not be required for such patients.

Biomechanics

Make your patient aware of the significance of abdominal breathing using the following calculation. Assuming that your patient is an adult with costosternal breathing and a relatively low resting respiratory rate of 12 breaths per minute, this means that she elevates her thorax against gravity 720 (12 × 60) times an hour, for 14 hours—in other words, 10,080 times a day. Per kilogram of thoracic weight, the patient with costosternal breathing therefore raises about 10 tons against gravity per day.

This work is performed by all the muscles surrounding the cervical spine and the muscles of mandibular elevation (masseter, temporalis, and medial pterygoid). The parafunctional breathing work of these muscles can lead to significant pain and dysfunction of the cervical spine, the shoulder–neck region, the head, the jaw, the larynx, and the brachial plexus.

For instance, in costosternal inspiration, the brachial plexus can be pinched between the anterior and medial scalene muscles (interscalene brachial plexus block), by the first rib, or the pectoralis minor muscle. This nerve compression can lead to reflex muscle tension in the shoulder girdle and arm. Furthermore, it can cause paresthesia in the arm and hand.

Retraining breathing can improve carpal tunnel symptoms

Patients with pronounced carpal tunnel symptoms (e.g., sleep disorders caused by paresthesia, electrical sensations in the hand on percussion of the carpal tunnel, and decreased nerve conduction velocites in this region) experience significant improvement or are even made symptom-free simply by retraining their breathing as described above.

Because of the attachment of the diaphragm to the vertebral bodies of the lumbar spine (L1–L4), the ribs (ribs 7–12), and the xiphoid process, a normal position and function of the lumbar and thoracic spine is only possible with relaxed abdominal breathing. Thus, it is not surprising that twisted vertebrae, especially around T6–T9, are often spontaneously repositioned with abdominal breathing.

Finally, the abdominal organs are pushed downward during diaphragmatic inspiration. This movement in response to the respiratory rhythm promotes the circulation and function of these organs.

5 Movement

5.1 Changing Seated Position

Test

Do you change your seated position from time to time? Sometimes unsupported, without a back rest (**Fig. 5.1 a**), sometimes supported with the pelvis pushed completely back to the back rest (**Fig. 5.1 b**), and sometimes, if the chair and your work permit, back to front in the chair (**Fig. 5.1 c**)?

Exercise

In your daily life, make sure that you change your seated posture from time to time: sometimes unsupported, without a back rest, sometimes supported with the pelvis pushed completely back to the back rest, and sometimes, if the chair and your work permit, back to front in the chair.

Troubleshooting

If your patient develops back problems because she sits for long periods on a seat without a back rest, she should see whether the change from unsupported sitting and sitting with the support of a back rest will provide any improvement.

Most people do well if they sit unsupported for two-thirds of the time and supported for one-third of the time. When the back muscles begin to feel tired, it is a good time to change from unsupported sitting to sitting with a support.

Before and After Comparison

For what percentage of extend periods of sitting does your patient alternate between sitting with and without a back rest?

Differential Diagnosis

Back pain can increase or decrease when leaning back against a back rest (**Fig. 5.1 b**).

If symptoms in the iliosacral region increase when the patient leans back, it is often because of a malalignment of an instable iliosacral joint (see "Biochmechanics" for this section). If this is the case, the symptoms subside as soon as and as long as the therapist manually corrects the malalignment while the patient remains in the same sitting position (**Fig. 5.1 b**).

If back pains that arise while sitting without a back rest subside when the patient leans back against a back rest, it can be because the back extensors have relaxed, cervical spine extension has decreased, or pressure on the disks, vertebral joints, and foramina has been relieved. The following tests help to determine which of these causes is re-

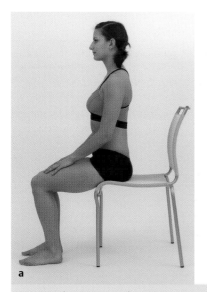
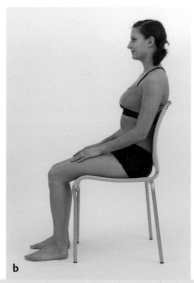
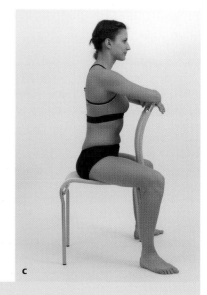

a   b   c

Fig. 5.1 Changing seated position.

sponsible for the symptoms associated with sitting unsupported:

- If *tensed back extensors* are the cause of pain when sitting unsupported, the pain will decrease as soon as the patient leans backward with a neutral spine, as in sitting with a balanced upper body when seated (p. 25) until her abdominal muscles contract. For differentiation, the back should not make contact with a back rest during this procedure.
- If the symptoms are caused by *hyperextension of the cervical spine* when sitting unsupported, they will decrease or increase with an isolated cervical spine flexion or extension, respectively. In this case, to correct the cervical spine posture efficaciously, it is essential to determine whether the hyperextension of the cervical spine is compensating for a deficit in thoracic extension mobility (p. 73).
- If the back pains are caused by a *pressure on the vertebral structures*, they may decrease or increase with longitudinal manual distraction or compression, respectively.

Biomechanics

Tipping the back rest together with the spinal segment resting on it to the horizontal lessens the pressure on the disks, facet joints, and intervertebral foramina. This is the case, on the one hand, because more and more upper body weight is being supported by the back rest. On the other hand, the postural muscles have to work less when the back rest is tipped backward, thus additionally decreasing the muscular compression of the spinal structures.

However, relaxation of the muscles also decreases their stabilizing effect on the spine and the iliosacral joints. The better stability of the iliosacral joints when sitting unsupported is due not only to better muscular stability, but also to more efficacious tension banding. Tension banding is based on the fact that the sacrum is pushed in an inferior direction by axial loading and thus tightens the stabilizing iliosacral ligaments.

Because of these advantages and disadvantages of a backward-inclined seated posture, alternation between supported and unsupported sitting makes sense. In addition, varying the seated posture prevents damage to individual spinal structures through unbalanced stress distribution.

If the patient tends to slouch when leaning against a high back rest, it is often helpful to use a slightly reclined back rest that ends just below the shoulder blades. This allows for the weight of the upper body to fall backward over the upper edge of the back rest. The resulting extension torque passively straightens the thoracic spine and, continuing down the kinetic chain, also the lumbar spine. This is balanced by increased tension in the abdominal muscles, which are also trained in this way. Because of their greater distance from the fulcrum in the vertebral body, the abdominal muscles do not have to contract as much for sta-

bilization of the spine as the back extensors do, and thus exert less compression on the spine.

5.2 Change of Position

Test

In the course of the day, do you alternate your position every 30 minutes between lying down, standing, walking, or sitting (**Fig. 5.2**)?

Exercise

In the course of the day, alternate your position every 30 minutes between lying down, standing, walking, or sitting.

Troubleshooting

Often it is impossible to alternate your position every 30 minutes because of the customary longer periods of sitting in school or at work. During these excessively long periods of sitting, the spine should be relieved of stress by the techniques of dynamic sitting and standing (p. 53).

For those who are bedridden, the position can be varied between lying supine, on the side, and prone. If only one of these positions is possible, the dynamic sitting exercises (p. 53) can be applied to the recumbent position.

Before and After Comparison

For what percentage of the day does your patient alternate her position every 30 minutes between lying down, standing, walking, or sitting?

Differential Diagnosis

In the case of a lumbar spinal stenosis, symptoms in the lumbar spine, hips, or legs typically increase while standing and subside immediately when the patient sits down. It can be determined whether the symptoms originate from the spinal stenosis or from the hip joints by means of passive end range hip flexion in the supine position.

End range hip flexion causes stenotic symptoms to decrease because it continues as lumbar flexion up the kinetic chain. Local hip symptoms, in contrast, tend to increase with end range hip flexion. With degenerative joint changes (coxarthrosis), femoroacetabular impingement, or an eccentric position of the femoral head, endgrade hip joint flexion is likely to cause a pinching pain in the groin. In case of less frequent tightness or inflammation of the hip extensor muscles, end range hip flexion will cause them to feel tight.

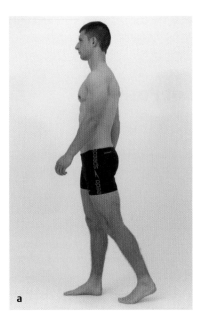
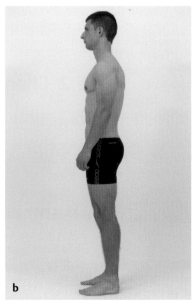
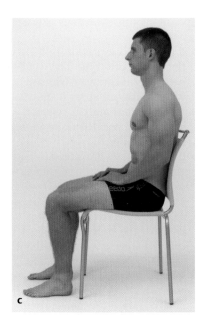
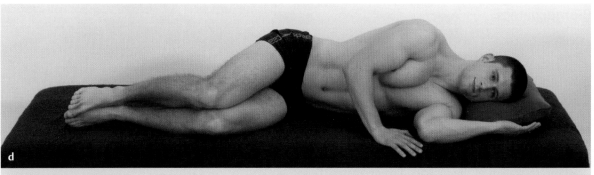

Fig. 5.2 Changes of position.

Biomechanics

A fundamental difference between sitting and standing is that, in standing, the thoracic and lumbar regions of the spine are automatically much more upright than in sitting. In a study of 107 office workers, the habitual thoracolumbar extension seen during sitting was 39% of maximal spinal extension. In standing, with the shoulders and buttocks touching the wall, it was 93% (Fischer 2013).

This large difference in flexion–extension means that the load on the spine is very different in sitting and standing:
• The spinal canal is narrowed with extension and widened with flexion. For this reason, it is not surprising that a lumbar spine stenosis creates many more symptoms during standing than sitting.

• When a person is slouched on a seat, the entire compression load of the lumbar spine is borne by the disks, whereas in the extended standing posture, a part of the compression load is also borne by the facet joints (Adams and Hutton 1980). For this reason, constant slouching while seated is a considerable risk factor for lumbar disk symptoms, whereas long periods of standing with a hyperextended lumbar spine overloads the facet joints.

The very different stress on the spine in sitting and standing makes a frequent alteration from sitting to standing an effective protection against unbalanced stress distribution.

5.3 Dynamic Sitting and Standing

Test

When you are sitting and standing, do you constantly keep moving around the midpoint of the balanced upper body posture when seated (p. 25) with neutral spinal curvature (p. 12), causing opposing muscle groups to alternately contract and relax in the process?

Exercise

When you are sitting and standing, keep moving around the midpoint of a balanced upper body posture with neutral spinal curvature (**Fig. 5.3**), causing the opposing muscle groups to alternately contract and relax in the process. A few options for a dynamic posture are described under the following alternative exercises.

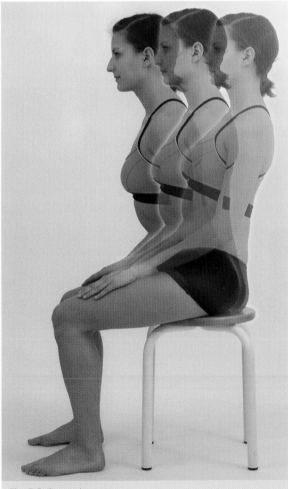

Fig. 5.3 Dynamic posture.

▶ **Alternative exercises for dynamic posture with a stabilized spine.** With a stabilized neutral spinal curvature (p. 12) you can alternately bend so far backward and so far forward (**Fig. 5.4**) that you feel how your abdominal and back muscles alternately tense and relax as described under "Balanced Upper Body when Seated" (p. 25). After a little practice, you will learn to feel this tensing and relaxing as a slight pressure or pull, even without using your fingers.

Awareness exercise: Muscle chains

Since your body will always orchestrate a synchronized contraction of numerous muscles as so-called muscle chains, you will learn to feel, after a time when you lean back, that the increased tension in your abdomen is accompanied by an increased tension in your larynx and face as well.

If you sit and lean to the right with your spine stabilized, you will feel your left ischial tuberosity rise (**Fig. 5.5 a**). If you stand and lean to the right with your spine stabilized, you will feel your left heel rise (**Fig. 5.5 b**). Regardless of whether you stand or sit, check whether you can feel how leaning to the right, with your spine stabilized, causes increased muscle tension on the left side of your body all the way from your waist to your face.

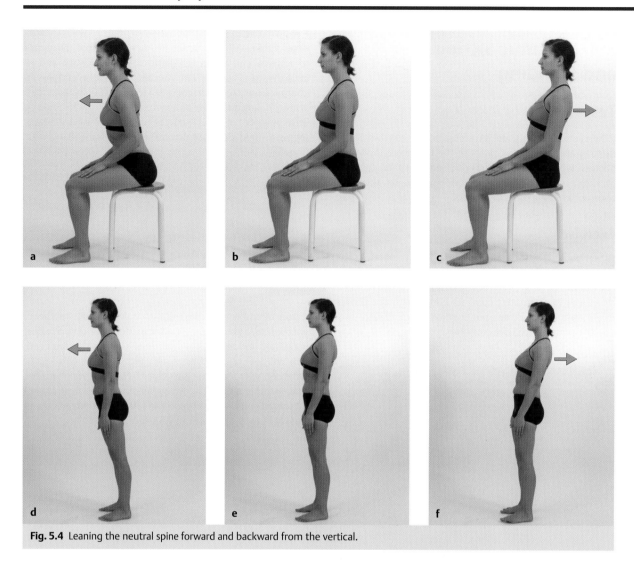

Fig. 5.4 Leaning the neutral spine forward and backward from the vertical.

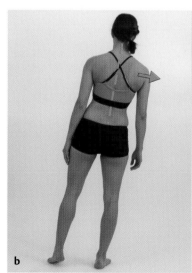

Fig. 5.5 Tensing the left trunk muscles with a stabilized spine: leaning the pelvis and thorax together to the right.

▶ **Alternative exercises for dynamic posture, with side bending, rotation, or flexion–extension of the spine**

Side bending
Hold your sternum steady in a forward and upward position while alternately raising the right and left sides of your pelvis (**Fig. 5.6**).

Rotation
Hold your sternum steady in a forward and upward position, while alternately advancing the right and left knee while sitting (**Fig. 5.7a**), or alternately advancing the right and left side of your pelvis while standing (**Fig. 5.7b**).

Flexion–extension
Flex and extend your spine by alternately slouching and then returning to an upright posture (**Fig. 5.8**). Notice how slouching causes your thorax to cave in and the chin to chest distance to increase, and how this reverses when you straighten up again.

▶ **More alternative exercises for dynamic standing**
- You can shift your weight from one foot to the other.
- You can alternately raise and lower your heels.
- You can draw horizontal figure 8 s with your hips.

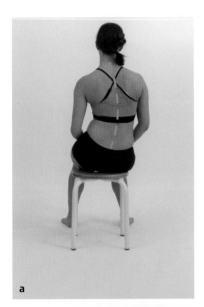
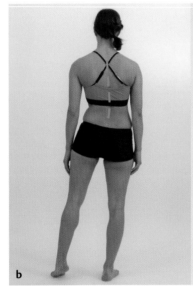

Fig. 5.6 Tensing of the muscles of the left side of the trunk by bending the lumbar spine to the left: raising the left side of the pelvis while keeping the thorax steady.

a

b

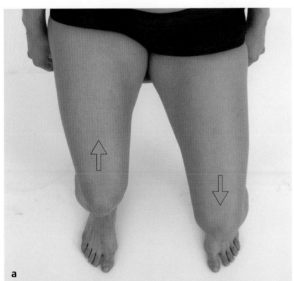
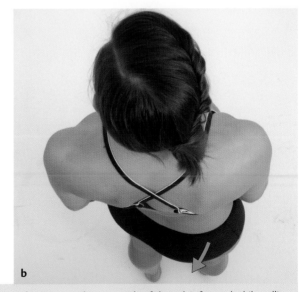

a

b

Fig. 5.7 Tensing a variety of abdominal and back muscles by rotating the spine: pushing one side of the pelvis forward while pulling the other side back, without moving the thorax.

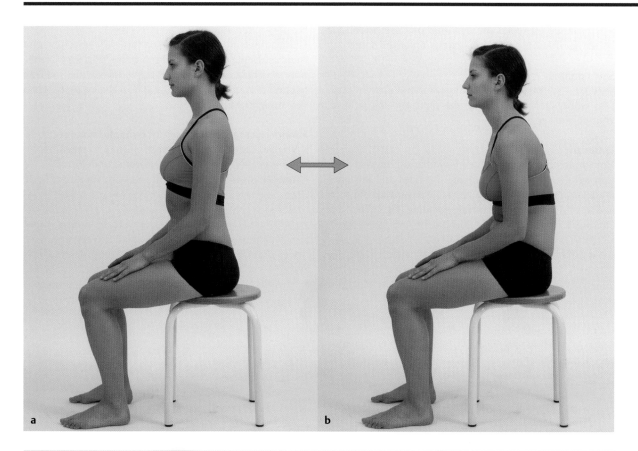

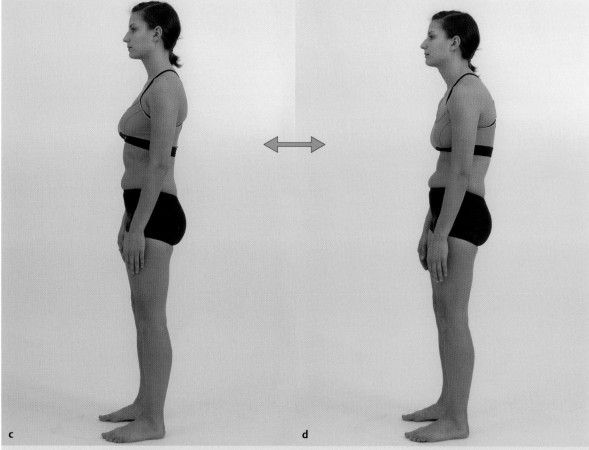

Fig. 5.8 Alternately slouch and straighten the spine.

Troubleshooting

An incorrect performance of the exercises due to poor co-ordination can usually be improved by having your patient exercise in front of a mirror.

Before and After Comparison

For what percentage of the time is your patient's sitting or standing position dynamic?

Differential Diagnosis

If raising the left side of the pelvis (see **Fig. 5.6**) causes pain on the left side of the lumbar spine, the source of the pain could be an irritated quadratus lumborum muscle or an impingement on the left side. The presence of a foraminal impingement can be determined by bending the spine to the left, starting with the head, without raising the pelvis. This narrows the left foramina without contraction of the left quadratus lumborum muscle. If this movement elicits the pain, the cause is a foraminal impingement or the rare case of an impingement between the iliac crest and lowest rib.

Biomechanics

Twomey and Taylor (1994) describe the following advantages of dynamic posture:
- Insufficient movement causes atrophy and degeneration of the articular cartilage and the underlying bones, especially under conditions of constant stress.
- Continuously maintaining the disks in an unchanged position is associated with pain and degeneration of the disks.
- Ligaments and cartilage react positively to movement.
- Movement is a prerequisite for fluid and nutrient transfer within the joints and the disks.

This may explain why using a lumbar support on a back rest that provides continuous passive extension and flexion of the lumbar spine decreases lumbar pain in seated individuals (Reinecke et al 1994).

6 Coordination

6.1 Sitting Up

Test

When you are lying in bed on your back and want to sit on the left edge of the bed, do you follow the steps shown in **Figs. 6.1**, **6.2**, **6.3**, **6.4**?

Exercise

In daily life, do you always move from lying on your back to sitting as described in **Figs. 6.1**, **6.2**, **6.3**, **6.4**? Try to progress smoothly through these steps in one flowing movement. When you lie down, follow the images in the opposite direction, starting with the bottom image (sitting) and move upward image by image to the top image (lying supine).

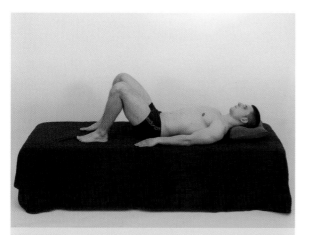

Fig. 6.1 First pull one heel close to your buttocks until you can comfortably place the sole of your foot on the bed, and then bring the other foot beside it.

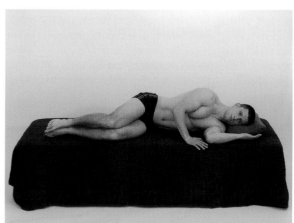

Fig. 6.2 Now turn onto your left side and support yourself on the bed with your right hand next to your left elbow.

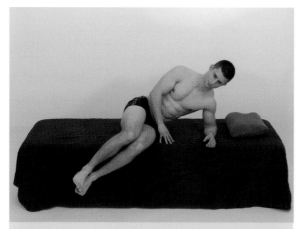

Fig. 6.3 Hang your lower legs over the edge of the bed and, finally, use your hands ...

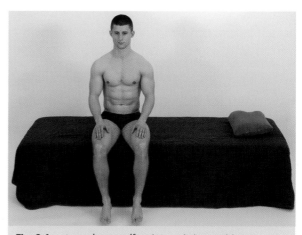

Fig. 6.4 ... to push yourself up into a sitting position.

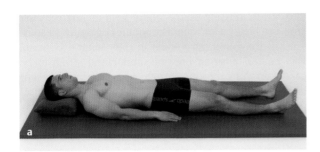

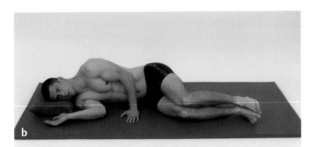

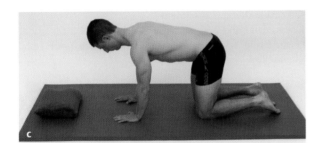

▶ **Alternative exercises.** If it is not possible to get out of bed at the side, the gentlest move for your back is to first turn onto your stomach, then rise onto your hands and knees, and finally to get off the bed on all fours at the free end.

The same is true for the upper level of bunk beds, where the ceiling is usually too low to permit sitting up.

If you are lying on the floor on your back and want to get up, you should also first turn onto your side. From there, support yourself on all fours and then on your knees. Next, put one leg forward and stand up (**Fig. 6.5**).

Troubleshooting

Back pain when moving from a supine to a sitting or a standing position can usually be avoided by doing so with a stabilized neutral spinal curvature (p. 23).

Repositioning the iliosacral joint

Pain in the iliosacral joint when lying supine and trying to turn onto the side can often be avoided if the patient holds one knee to her abdomen with both hands as described under "Differential Diagnosis" below.

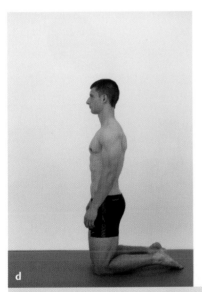

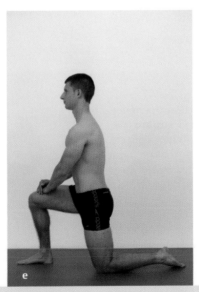

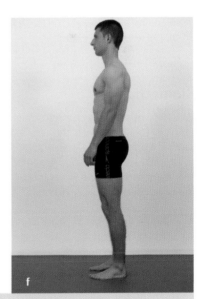

Fig. 6.5 Progression from lying on the back, to lying on the side, to being on all fours, to kneeling, kneeling with one foot forward, and standing.

Before and After Comparison

For what percentage of the time does the patient make the transition from lying on her back to sitting and vice versa through the intermediate position of lying on her side?

Differential Diagnosis

If your patient's attempt to turn from her back to her side causes iliosacral pain, the cause is usually twisting or instability in the iliosacral joint. More rarely, the cause is instability in the lower lumbar vertebrae. To distinguish between the lumbar spine and the sacroiliac joint as the source of the pain, the patient should keep one knee pulled all the way to her abdomen while turning onto her side. Symptoms that originate in the lumbar spine will not vary a great deal in regard to whether the left or the right knee is pulled up to the abdomen. But if the symptoms are originating in the sacroiliac joint, it does make a difference. If an ilium is rotated posteriorly, it can be expected that the pain caused by transitioning from supine to lying on the side will be less if the contralateral knee is held to the abdomen. If the ilium is rotated anteriorly, on the other hand, it is usually more helpful to hold the ipsilateral knee to the abdomen while turning.

Flexion versus extension

Lumbar spine pain that is due to an injury to the posterior annulus of a disk and sets in when standing up usually decreases if a lordotic curvature of the lumbar spine is maintained during the movement. Pain caused by foraminal impingement, on the other hand, can be reduced with more flexion.

Biomechanics

When the upper body is raised straight up from the supine position to sitting with the legs extended forward, the lumbar spine is flexed unless a conscious effort is made to keep it extended. In this flexed position, the compressive load on the spine is no longer carried by the facet joints, but entirely by the disks.

In addition, in the initial phase of raising the upper body straight up, support from the arms is typically absent, while at the same time, the lever arm of the upper body weight is maximal in relation to the lumbar spine. This creates significant torque in the lumbar spine that must be compensated by a correspondingly strong contraction of the stomach muscles. The muscle tension required to support the upper body close to the horizontal can compress the disks with a force that is many times greater than the load of the upper body's weight in a standing position (Wilke et al 1999). Thus, this muscle tension—especially when the lumbar spine is flexed—can overload the disk to the point of rupture.

In contrast, in rising from a lateral position (**Fig. 6.2**), the arms can be used for support from the beginning. In addition, all the joints can remain in their neutral position. This neutral position prevents nonneutral stress to be passed on along the kinetic chain. In contrast, insufficient hamstring flexibility leads to compensatory non-neutral flexion of the lumbar spine, when raising the upper body into a long sitting position.

6.2 Balance

Test

When you are putting on and taking off your shoes and socks, can you keep your balance and stabilize your spine while standing (**Fig. 6.6**)?

To check this, stand on a hard, even surface and place your right foot on your left thigh. You have passed the test if you succeed in doing the following:

1. You can bend forward with a stabilized neutral spinal curvature (p. 23) until your hands reach your right shoe.

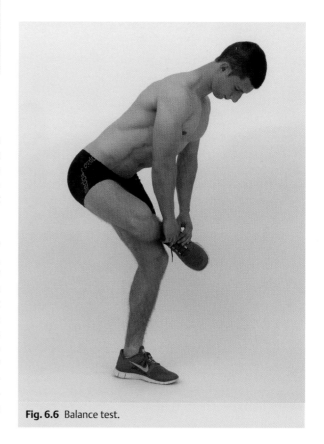

Fig. 6.6 Balance test.

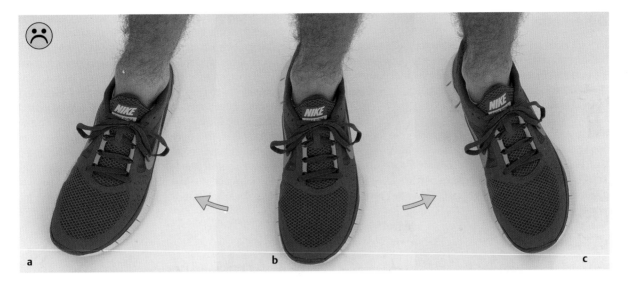

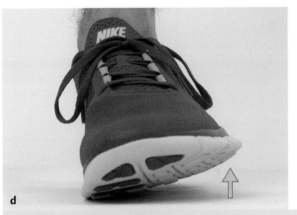

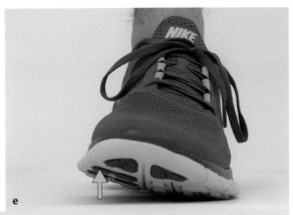

Fig. 6.7 You have failed the test if the left foot slips (**a, b**) or rises from the floor on either side (**d, e**).

2. In this position, you can take off your right shoe and right sock and put them on again with so little loss of balance that your left shoe neither slips nor rises from the floor at either the outer or the inner side (**Figs. 6.6 and 6.7**).
3. You can repeat this with your eyes closed.

Exercise

In daily life, try to put on and take off your shoes and socks as described above while standing. If this is easy with your eyes open, try it with closed eyes as well.

▶ **Alternative exercises.** If even the exercise with open eyes is too difficult, the patient can start with easier balance exercises. One example is standing on one foot. If this is also too difficult, the patient can start by placing her feet close together or by walking heel to toe along a line on the floor, imagining it to be a tightrope.

Troubleshooting

If even the balance exercise with open eyes is too difficult, the patient can start with the easier alternative exercises described above.

Improving limited calf flexibility (p. 103) immediately makes the balance reaction noticeably easier.

Before and After Comparison

For what percentage of the time can the patient keep her balance while putting on and taking off her shoes and socks as described in the "Test" section on p. 60? Can she do this only with her eyes open or does she succeed with her eyes closed as well?

Differential Diagnosis

If there is no visual input because the eyes are closed, the balance reaction depends more heavily on positional information from the inner ear and proprioceptors. Thus, the inner ear and proprioception can be better tested and trained with the eyes closed.

If balance improves through mobilization of a limited talocrural dorsiflexion, the impediment was mechanical. Calf flexibility (p. 103) is also required for dorsiflexion. Testing calf flexibility is therefore particularly important in patients whose balance problems are most pronounced while squatting.

Biomechanics

Balance training improves the ability of the muscles to contract at the right moment and to the right extent. This protects both the joints and the muscles themselves from unnecessary stress.

In addition to a sense of equilibrium, balance also requires that the joints are free to move as planned by the motor cortex. If, for instance, calf flexibility (p. 103) is limited, the center of gravity of the body can no longer be positioned over the anterior part of the area of support. Since our balance requires the body's center of gravity to be over the area of support, the reduced area of support also limits the possibility of a balance reaction in an anterior direction. The problem becomes more acute in the squatting position because squatting tenses the soleus muscle. As a result, it is easier for the patient to tip over backward. Usually, patients try to compensate for this kind of dorsal extension deficit through a plantar flexion of the talocrural joint, that is by lifting the heel and standing only on the balls of their feet. This makes it possible to shift the weight forward. But this move comes at the cost of exchanging a large area of support, the sole of the foot, for a much smaller area of support, the ball of the foot, so that the patient does not gain much stability in this way and still feels insecure.

6.3 Arm Swing

Test

When you are walking at a pace of two steps per second, do your arms swing along so freely that your hands swing completely past your thighs (**Fig. 6.8**)? Starting at a pace of two steps per second, the left hand should swing forward (**Fig. 6.8**, ①) and backward (**Fig. 6.8**, ②) completely past the left thigh (**Fig. 6.8**, ③). The forward swing should pass distinctly forward of the thigh (**Fig. 6.8**, ①), and the back-

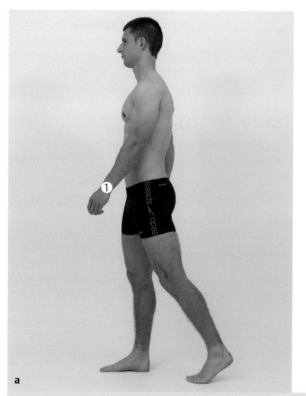 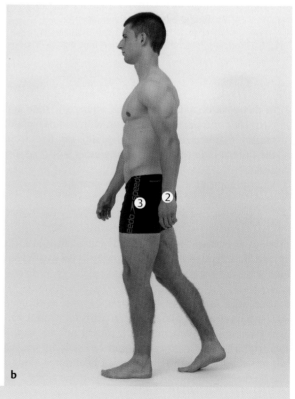

Fig. 6.8 Swinging the arms.

ward swing should extend barely behind the thigh (**Fig. 6.8**, ②). At the same time, the right hand should swing past the right thigh in the opposite direction. At a more rapid walking pace, the arm's swinging motion is wider. The left arm swings forward when the right leg moves forward, and vice versa. The arms need not be consciously swung. They swing along automatically when they are left loose and not slowed down by a bag or a broad pelvis.

Exercise

Try to let your arms swing along freely when you are walking. Make sure that both your arms swing equally far.

Troubleshooting

Bags carried by hand or over a shoulder hinder the swing of the ipsilateral arm. For this reason, carrying a backpack on the back is a better choice. To avoid tension in the upper trapezius, it should be a backpack with a hip belt so that the weight does not hang on the shoulders but is carried by the pelvis. Another impediment to a free swing of the ipsilateral arm is a protracted shoulder. Depending on the cause, the protraction may be corrected by improving shoulder mobility (p. 78), rotational mobility (p. 90), or shoulder blade and triceps muscle strength (p. 120).

Before and After Comparison

For what percentage of the time do your patient's arms swing along freely and evenly while walking?

Differential Diagnosis

If the right arm deviates markedly toward the midline on the forward swing, this can be the result of protraction of the right shoulder or left rotation of the entire thorax.

Protraction of the shoulder can be recognized by the fact that the distance between the scapula and the spinal column is greater ipsilaterally than contralaterally. Habitual protraction of the shoulder is more likely to affect the side of the dominant hand and is also usually associated with a lowered shoulder that disappears immediately with corrective retraction. The dominant side is more likely to be affected because it is used for reaching forward more frequently than the nondominant side. Over time, the body adapts to a habitual protraction with tense and short scapular protractors and glenohumeral external rotators, while the muscles that retract the scapula elongate and atrophy. If and to what extent this has taken place can be determined and corrected with the tests and exercises for shoulder mobility (p. 78), rotational mobility (p. 90), and shoulder blade and triceps muscle strength (p. 120).

Biomechanics

An effective push-off in walking is associated with pelvic and spinal rotation. This rotation is first braked by the arm swing and stored as elastic energy in the spine, to be discharged again as a driving force at the start of the next step, as with a wound-up rubber band.

If the arm swing is absent, this elastic braking and driving energy is also absent and must be compensated for by increased muscle work. This additional work leads to tensions and blocks the natural gait pattern.

6.4 Hip Extension

Test

1. In walking, do both of your hips extend so freely that your knee (**Fig. 6.9**, ①) moves effortlessly behind the hip bone in the stance phase (**Fig. 6.9**, ②)?
2. Do you allow your hip to move back along with your knee during the stance phase (**Fig. 6.9**, blue arrow), so that when you freeze mid-walk with your left leg one step behind and look down at your pelvis, you see how it is turned a little to the left (**Fig. 6.9**) rather than facing straight forward.

Exercise

In walking, let your knees swing through far to the back under your body (**Fig. 6.9**, ①). Also allow your pelvis, together with the ipsilateral knee, to swing somewhat backward (**Fig. 6.9**, ②). If you feel that hip extension is less free on one side, try to "copy" the freer feeling of the other side. Also check whether hip extension seems easier immediately after exercising hip extension mobility (p. 109). If yes, the hip extension mobility exercise would be a good preparation for longer walks during which you should consciously allow your newly gained hip extension to take place.

Troubleshooting

If the hip extension and posterior rotation of the ipsilateral pelvis in the transverse plane described in the exercise are restricted, you should check whether there is a deficit in hip extension mobility (p. 109), calf flexibility (p. 103), or rotational mobility (p. 90). When a deficit in these areas is improved, the hip extension in walking partly improves spontaneously. Sometimes, however, a patient retains her old movement pattern and must be reminded to use her newly achieved freedom of movement.

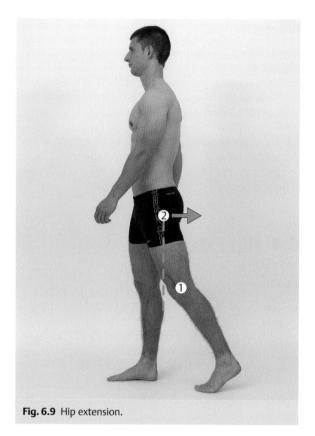

Fig. 6.9 Hip extension.

The hip swing (**Fig. 6.9**, ②) generates the energy for effective forward movement. Therefore, it should match the pace. In sprinting, the movement must be large and strong, and in slow walking, it must be more modest. If the gait with the newly learned hip swing (**Fig. 6.9**, ②) seems unnatural, this is usually because it is exaggerated for the walking pace or because the counterbalancing arm swing (p. 62) is too small. A natural gait may then be achieved by adjusting the arm swing and the walking pace to match the hip swing, or vice versa.

Before and After Comparison

In walking, how many degrees does the long axis of the thigh rotate backward from the vertical during the stance phase? Alternatively, it is also possible to compare how far backward the knee moves behind a plumb line through the hip bone (**Fig. 6.9**).

Differential Diagnosis

It can be determined whether restricted hip extension in walking is caused by an elastic resistance or whether hip extension mobility is actually free and is only not used because of a parafunctional movement pattern, by testing hip extension mobility (p. 109), calf flexibility (p. 103), and rotational mobility (p. 90). If one or more of these tests is positive, the respective elastic resistances are limit-

ing hip extension. On the other hand, if mobility in these areas is free, the cause is primarily a parafunctional movement pattern. Quite often, natural flexibility and movement patterns are lost due to prolonged, monotonous, and static sitting in school, at work, and increasingly also during leisure time.

Hypertonicity of the iliopsoas muscle that hinders free hip extension mobility (p. 109) is most often caused by irritation in the area of the lumbar spine, hip joint, intestine, or by an inguinal hernia.

- Irritation of the lumbar spine caused by compression is intensified by end range movements and axial compression; it decreases noticeably under traction. The duration of compression necessary to provoke the symptoms depends on the level of irritability. Indications of irritability are provided by testing the range of motion and, in the medical history, noting how long it takes a certain stress to provoke the symptoms.
- If the hip joint is irritated, the symptoms are intensified in step 1 of inner thigh flexibility (p. 106). With more intense irritation of the hip joint, the muscle tension tends to increase rather than decrease in the course of the hip extension mobility exercise (p. 109).
- If the increased tone of the iliopsoas muscle is caused by an intestinal irritation, the resulting symptoms are relieved noticeably after a large bowel movement.
- Finally, irritation caused by an inguinal hernia is typically increased when the intra-abdominal pressure increases in response to activities such as coughing or lifting.

Biomechanics

A free hip extension continues as a rotation in the spine, where it is an important element of the natural gait pattern. This requires the iliopsoas muscle to be able to relax and be flexible, which also unloads all the joints lying between its origin and attachment, namely the joints and disks of the lumbar vertebrae as well as the ipsilateral iliosacral and hip joint. In addition, the wide hip extension movement in walking distributes the weight over a wide surface of the femoral head and thus helps to protect it from osteoarthritis.

6.5 Eye Muscle Coordination

Test

Can you move your eyes, slowly and evenly, in a large circle, as though from hour to hour on a clock face, without a feeling of tension (**Fig. 6.10**), without skipping an hour, while your facial expression, your head, and your lower jaw remain so relaxed that they do not move along with your eyes?

Start with a clockwise circular motion of the eyes and repeat the same procedure counterclockwise. Leave yourself 12 seconds to complete the circle, that is, 1 second for each hour on the imaginary clock face. If you are not sure whether your eye movement is slow and regular, ask someone you are face to face with to control your eye movement.

Exercise

Move your eyes in a circle, as described under "Test" (p. 65), very slowly and regularly, without skipping an hour, with your facial expression, head, and lower jaw so relaxed that they do not move along with your eyes. If you do not succeed in covering some part of the circle with your eye movement, or do so only with an unpleasant feeling of tension in the area of your eyes, you should move your eyes back and forth only in this area of the circle until the movement is rounder and the tension disappears.

▶ **Alternative exercise.** You can increase the challenge if you combine the eye muscle coordination exercise with the exercise for leg, back, and cranial nerve mobility (p. 98) or the arm nerve mobility exercise (p. 83). This combination is useful only if and for as long as it makes eye muscle coordination appreciably more difficult.

Troubleshooting

If the exercise causes an unpleasant feeling of tension in the area of the eyes that does not disappear with practice, the following tests and exercises should be used to detect and resolve possible mechanical impediments. If one of the following tests is positive, have your patient do the corresponding exercise and then repeat the eye muscle coordination test. If the circular eye motion can now be done without tension, you have found and solved the problem.
- Do all relaxation exercises simultaneously (pp. 39 – 49)
- Leg, back, and cranial nerve mobility (p. 98)
- Arm nerve mobility (p. 83)
- Thoracic extension mobility (p. 73)

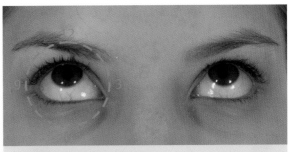

Fig. 6.10 Eye muscle coordination.

Dissociation

If your patient does not pass the test because she moves her jaw or her head, this movement is probably occurring in the form of an ipsilateral lateral movement of the lower jaw or an ipsilateral rotation of the cervical spine. These habitual en-bloc movement patterns can be resolved with dissociated contralateral movements. That is, the patient looks to the right with her eyes, without moving her head, while her lower jaw is displaced to the left (**Fig. 6.11**).

Before and After Comparison

Is the eye movement rounder, with less tension or associated movement of facial expression, lower jaw, and head?

Differential Diagnosis

Often headaches caused by unbalanced eye muscles are intensified by reading. Looking out the window of a moving train is also particularly stressful for the eye muscles. The nystagmus that arises naturally from this activity can also overexert dysfunctional eye muscles and thus trigger a headache.

If a restricted neurodynamic contributes to tension in the eyes during the eye muscle coordination exercise, the feeling of tension will increase in combination with the leg, back, and cranial nerve mobility exercise (p. 98) or the arm nerve mobility exercise (p. 83).

Neck muscles that compensate for unbalanced eye muscles relax immediately upon restoration of eye muscle balance.

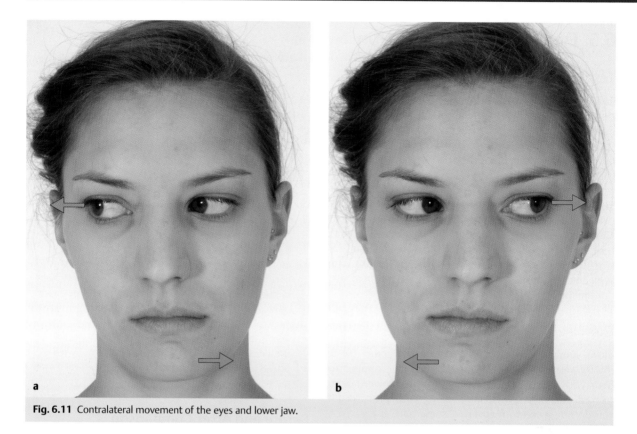

Fig. 6.11 Contralateral movement of the eyes and lower jaw.

Biomechanics

If we keep our eyes focused on an object while turning our head a little to the left, our eye muscles must move our eye just as far to the right in order to keep the object in view. Because of this closely coordinated muscle control of the cervical spine and eye, good eye muscle coordination relaxes not only the eyes, but automatically also the neck muscles. Conversely, relaxed neck muscles promote relaxed vision.

Dural tension

The dura mater ensheathes the optic nerve. For this reason, tension in the dura mater can be mechanically transmitted to the eyes and contribute to tension in the eye muscles or the feeling that one cannot see clearly, even though the ophthalmological findings are negative.

Additional Tests
and Exercises

7 Mobility

Some basic principles must be kept in mind in mobility training.

▶ **Tension**

> ### First feeling of tension
>
> When your patient experiences the first, slight feeling of tension, she should stop and hold this position. It is this position that determines whether or not the test was passed. The exercise consists of letting the tension resolve in this position, without any further movement.

Help your patient exercise successfully by instructing her to focus on relaxing until she actually feels how the tension decreases. After this, if she has the time and motivation, she can move further toward the test goal until she encounters the next slight resistance.

Training the mental ability to relax specific muscles is an important requirement for healthy mobility. For this reason, your patient should always build up only as much tension as she can relax. Depending on how well she has learned conscious relaxation, complete relaxation can take between 30 seconds and 5 minutes. If your patient has not been able to relax after 2 minutes, she should try with more concentration, less tension, or take a short break before trying again.

> ### Muscle guarding
>
> In the rare cases in which muscle tension cannot be resolved in this way, you should stop the exercise and investigate whether the muscle tension is protecting irritated, injured, or overloaded tissues. The exercise should then only be continued after the cause has been eliminated.

Common mistake

The most common mistake in mobility exercises is that patients do not go to the first, slight tension, as recommended, but to the pain threshold. This creates a reflex increase in tension in the stretched muscle, to guard against further stretching. This muscle guarding prevents any improvement in mobility. In addition, stretching with excessive tension increases the likelihood of straining the muscle and its tendon. For this reason, patients should be repeatedly reminded only to go as far as the first, slight tension.

▶ **Order of exercises.** The following mobility tests and exercises are arranged according to body regions, from top to bottom. Stretches of structures in the back of the leg are followed by stretches for anterior structures of the leg. When treating a patient, you should, however, start with the clinically most relevant test rather than maintaining the order of going from top to bottom and back to front. You can determine the clinically most relevant test on the basis of your clinical experience or with the help of the navigator (p. 146).

▶ **Left and right.** Mobility tests that are performed individually for each side of the body are described for only one side (the left side) for reasons of brevity and clarity. Naturally, they are also to be performed analogously on the other side. If your patient passes one of these tests on the left side and does not pass it on the right side, she will need to do the exercise only on the right side.

▶ **Chair height and gym mat.** Seated exercises assume a seat height at which the hips are positioned a little higher than the knees (p. 28). Doing exercises in which your patient kneels or lies on the floor on a gym mat is more comfortable, and thus facilitates relaxation and efficacious exercising.

▶ **Time of day.** Since mobility generally increases during the course of an active day, it is easier to pass the mobility tests in the evening. But so that healthy mobility is already accessible in the morning, it is ideal if your patient remains or becomes so mobile that she can already pass the mobility tests 1 hour after rising.

▶ **Distance from test objective**

> ### Measurement units
>
> In the mobility tests, the distance from the test objective is measured in centimeters or finger widths (p. 179).

Measurement in finger widths has the advantage that it is particularly quick and simple. However, it assumes that re-examination will be done by the same therapist or another therapist with the same finger width. Moreover, it assumes that a therapist who measures with both left and right hands has equally wide fingers on both hands.

Measurement in centimeters allows for a more accurate statistical analysis and avoids errors due to inconsistent finger width. Thus measurement in centimeters is advisable if a patient will be measured by more than one therapist or if the results will be used for statistical analysis.

7.1 Chin Tuck Mobility

▶ **Starting position.** Stand with your back to a wall, your feet a shoe width apart (see **Fig. 3.26**), and your heels one foot length away from the wall. Lean against the wall with your buttocks and shoulders and bend your knees slightly. Place one hand on your neck right underneath your skull. Now tip your head so far forward that you can see the front of your body (feet, chest, or abdomen) (**Fig. 7.1**, ①) and hold it in this "double chin" position.

Test

Can you keep your neck in a double chin position and push it so far back that one finger knuckle (**Fig. 7.1**, ②) touches the wall, without experiencing pain or tension in your neck and without losing sight of the front of your body (**Fig. 7.1**, ①)?

Exercise

Push your neck back until you feel the onset of tension in your neck. Remain in this position until the tension resolves.

> **Without a hand**
>
> The hand at the neck is only used for the test. For the exercise, your arms should hang loosely by your sides (**Fig. 7.2**). This facilitates concentration on the intended extension of the cervical spine.

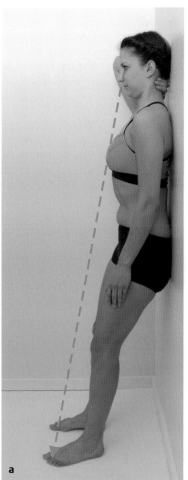
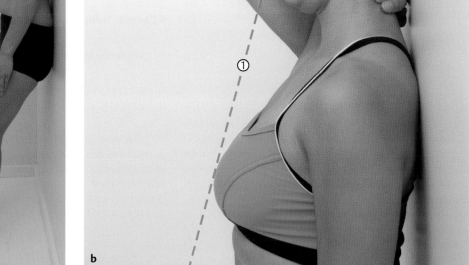

Fig. 7.1 Chin tuck mobility test.

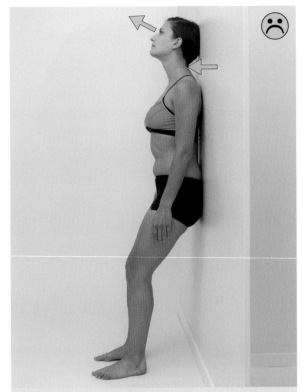

Fig. 7.2 Doing the exercise incorrectly with a hyperextended cervical spine.

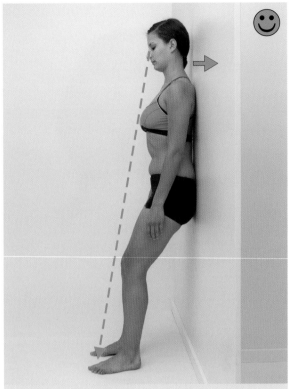

Fig. 7.3 Performing the exercise correctly with the chest, abdomen, or feet in view.

So that you do not hyperextend your cervical spine while doing this exercise (**Fig. 7.2**), it is important that you always keep the front of your body in view. Always check: Can I still see the front of my body (**Fig. 7.3**)?

▶ **Alternative exercise.** Chin tuck mobility can also be practiced without a wall. To do this, place a fist against the front of your voice box (**Fig. 7.4**). Next, tip your head forward until your chin makes contact with your fist, and then slide your chin backward on your fist until you feel a slight tension in your neck (**Fig. 7.5**). As soon as this movement has become routine and can be repeated reliably, it suffices to just imagine the fist.

Troubleshooting

If chin tuck mobility is restricted, patients often try to push their head toward the wall rather than their cervical spine. This leads to hyperextension of the cervical spine and prevents the desired elongation of the cervical spine. For this reason, patients must be repeatedly reminded to keep the front of their body in view.

Common mistake

You should make your patient aware of the following important difference: The head is not required to touch the wall, during either the test or the exercise. It is the neck and not the head that must be pushed backward toward the wall.

If the tension still does not diminish over the course of the exercise, the following tests and exercises should be used to detect and resolve possible mechanical impediments. If one of the following tests is positive, have your patient do the corresponding exercise and then repeat the chin tuck mobility exercise. If the tension resolves, you have found and eliminated the mechanical impediment.

- Repeat the exercise with less tension while simultaneously doing all the relaxation exercises (pp. 39–49)
- Thoracic extension mobility (p. 73)
- Rotational mobility (p. 90)
- Arm nerve mobility (p. 83)
- Leg, back, and cranial nerve mobility (p. 98)
- Eye muscle coordination (p. 65)

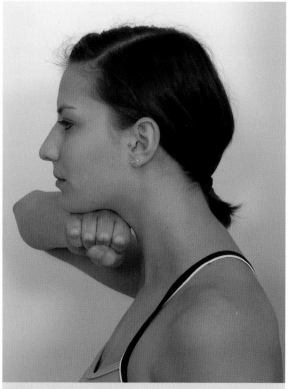

Fig. 7.4 Rest your chin on your fist in front of your voice box …

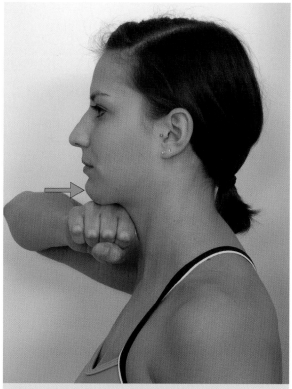

Fig. 7.5 … and slide your chin backward on your fist.

Before and After Comparison

At the narrowest point, how great is the distance between the wall and the patient's fingers on her neck (**Fig. 7.6**)?

Differential Diagnosis

If tensions or other symptoms are not resolved even after doing the exercises described in "Troubleshooting" in this section, instability of the transverse ligament (C1) or the dens (C2) must be ruled out. To do this, the therapist places one hand on the patient's forehead while the patient proceeds with the chin tuck mobility exercise until slight symptoms set in. The therapist holds the thumb and index finger of his free hand in a key pinch position and gives the C2 spinous process a slight forward push while holding the patient's head in position with his hand on her forehead. A decrease in symptoms with this maneuver indicates instability between C1 and C2. In this case, the exercise should only be continued after medical confirmation of suboccipital stability, and should remain within a range that does not provoke or intensify the symptoms, as is true for all exercises.

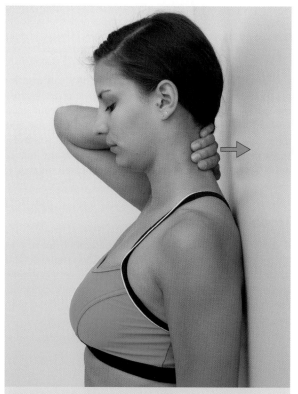

Fig. 7.6 The distance between the fingers and the wall.

Biomechanics

Painful, limited cervical spine rotation due to ipsilateral impingement in the intervertebral foramina is a common complaint. In this case rotating the spine into the restriction is usually counterproductive since it intensifies the impingement and the resulting symptoms. Indirect practice of the chin tuck mobility exercise alone or as part of the thoracic extension mobility exercise (**Fig. 7.9**) on the other hand usually produces a pronounced improvement in cervical spine rotation in the before and after comparison. This positive effect can be explained as follows:

- In the chin tuck mobility exercise, the upper and middle cervical spine is flexed. This flexion separates the facet joints, widens the intervertebral foramina, and stretches the capsule of the facet joints. When the capsule is loosened in this manner, the compression of the intervertebral foramina in end range rotation is reduced.

- Contraction of the anterior neck muscles leads to antagonistic relaxation of the extensors. This relaxation usually persists after the exercise has been completed and decompresses the foramina as well.

- When the head is positioned over and not in front of the shoulders, the facet joints are brought into a physiological position. At the same time, the neck muscles can relax better because the head is balanced in this position.

7.2 Thoracic Extension Mobility

▶ **Starting position.** Stand with your back to a wall, with your heels the length of your foot away from the wall, and your feet separated by the width of a shoe. Lean against the wall with your buttocks and shoulders, and bend your knees slightly. Tip your pelvis so that your lumbar spine is pressed against the wall (**Fig. 7.7**, ①). Finally, interlace your fingers at the back of your neck just below your skull,

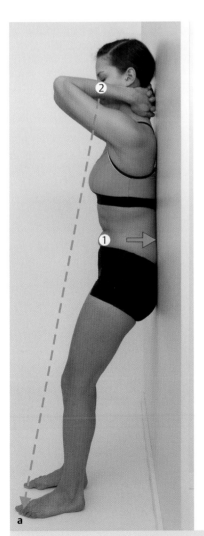
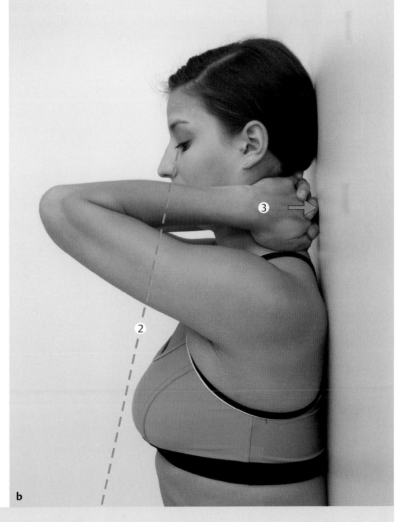

Fig. 7.7 Thoracic extension mobility test.

tip your head so far forward that you can see the front of your body (feet, chest, or abdomen) (**Fig. 7.7**, ②), and hold this "double chin" position. Make sure you avoid the most common mistake of losing this position by hyperextending your neck and losing sight of the front of your body (**Fig. 7.8**) while doing the following test and exercise.

Test

Can you keep your lumbar spine pressed against the wall (see **Fig. 7.7**, ①) while you push your neck backward until a knuckle of your interlaced fingers touches the wall (**Fig. 7.7**, ③), and you can still see the front of your body (**Fig. 7.7**, ②)—all without pain or tension in your neck and back?

Exercise

Keep your lumbar spine pressed against the wall and push your neck back until you feel the onset of tension in your neck or back. Remain in this position until the tension resolves.

The interlaced fingers at the neck are needed only for the test. For the exercise, your arms should hang loosely by your sides (**Fig. 7.9**). This facilitates concentration on the intended extension of the thoracic spine.

So that you do not hyperextend your cervical spine while exercising (see **Fig. 7.8**), it is important that you always maintain the front of your body in view. Always check: can I still see the front of my body (**Fig. 7.9**)?

▶ **Alternative exercise.** If you cannot push your lumbar spine to the wall (**Fig. 7.9**) or if thoracic extension does not improve over the course of the exercise, you can try the alternative exercise lying on your back with your knees bent. If the cervical spine is hyperextended in the supine position because of limited thoracic extension mobility (**Fig. 7.10**), the head should be supported with a pillow of appropriate height (**Fig. 7.11**).

When doing the exercise in the supine position, your arms should be placed next to your body. In this starting position, the cervical spine should be pushed toward the floor as far as possible without an increase in symptoms. Then try to see how far toward the floor you can push your lumbar spine without resulting pain and without increasing the distance between your cervical spine and the floor. As in all mobility exercises, this position should not cause pain or other symptoms, and it should be held until a reduction in tension or an increase in mobility is felt.

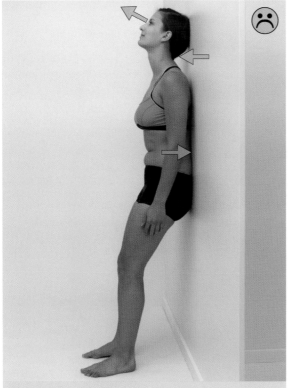

Fig. 7.8 Performing the exercise incorrectly with a hyperextended cervical spine.

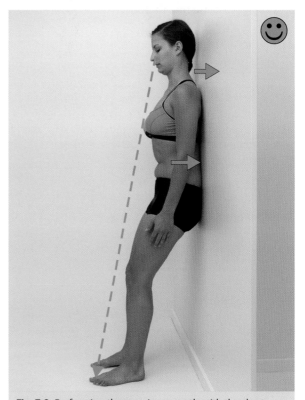

Fig. 7.9 Performing the exercise correctly with the chest, abdomen, or feet in view.

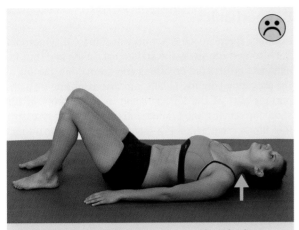

Fig. 7.10 Performing the exercise incorrectly with a hyper-extended cervical spine.

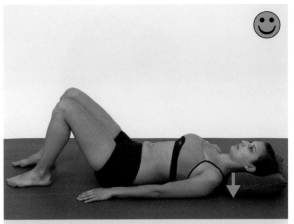

Fig. 7.11 Performing the exercise correctly with the chin close to the chest.

Exercising in the supine position is much simpler because thoracic extension works with rather than against gravity. In addition, for most people, coordination is easier in this position. As soon as the exercise can be done in supine position without problems, it should again be tried standing, so that the patient learns to straighten her spine any time she is in the vertical position. For the same reason, the supine position is not an alternative to the standing test (see **Fig. 7.7**). The test in the vertical position is more specific to spinal loading during daily activities and is meant to check whether a healthy, unrestricted extension of the spine is possible under these conditions.

Troubleshooting

Initially, patients often lack the coordination required for pressing their lumbar spine against the wall. Instead of tipping the pelvis, as required, they lift their heels and straighten their knees. In this case, patients need to be instructed to tip their pelvis by contracting their buttocks and abdominal muscles without raising their heels or straightening their knees.

Even more frequently, patients hyperextend their cervical spine during the exercise (see **Fig. 7.8**). This prevents the thoracic extension and cervical elongation for which the exercise is intended. For this reason, the patient must be repeatedly reminded to keep the front of her body in view (see **Fig. 7.9**).

> ### Common mistake
>
> In this exercise, the head does not need to touch the wall because it is the neck and not the head that must be pushed backward toward the wall.

If the tension still does not diminish over the course of the exercise, the following tests and exercises should be used to detect and resolve possible mechanical impediments to thoracic spine extension. If one of the following tests is positive, have your patient do the corresponding exercise and then repeat the thoracic extension mobility exercise. If the tension now has diminished you have found and eliminated the mechanical impediment.

- Repeat the exercise with less tension while simultaneously doing all the relaxation exercises (p. 39)
- Rotational mobility (p. 90)
- Leg, back, and cranial nerve mobility (p. 98)
- Alternative exercises in the supine position (**Fig. 7.11**).
- Manual mobilization of hypomobile thoracic vertebrae and ribs

Before and After Comparison

At the narrowest point, how great is the distance between the wall and the knuckles of the interlaced fingers at the patient's neck (**Fig. 7.12**)?

The patient is asked to keep her lumbar spine in contact with the wall during the test. If the patient, however, is unable to touch her lumbar spine against the wall to start with (see "starting position," p. 73), the distance between the wall and the lumbar spine ist added on. So, for example, if the distance between the knuckles at the neck and the wall is 2 cm in the test, and there is an additional space of 1 cm between the lumbar spine and the wall, the total of 3 cm is recorded.

Differential Diagnosis

Thoracic spine extension can be limited not only by hypomobility of the thoracic facet joints, but also by increased muscle tone in the abdominal muscles or the diaphragm. If increased muscle tone in the abdominal muscles or the diaphragm is causing the limitation, thoracic extension can be improved by manual trigger point treatment of the affected muscles or by doing the rotational mobility (p. 90) and abdominal breathing (p. 47) exercises.

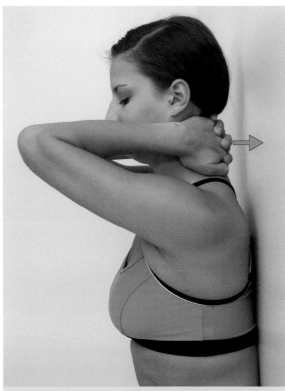

Fig. 7.12 The distance between the knuckles and the wall.

Biomechanics

An erect thoracic spine not only avoids local symptoms, but also decompresses the abdominal cavity, and thus facilitates unrestricted breathing and normal functioning of the abdominal organs. Finally, thoracic extension is an important part of the kinetic chain in movements of the shoulder, cervical spine, and lumbar spine. For this reason, free thoracic extension is a requirement for normal function in these regions.

> **Thoracic spine–shoulder study**
>
> Limited thoracic extension increases the likelihood of glenohumeral impingement (Betz et al 2005).

7.3 Back Muscle Flexibility

▶ **Starting position.** Kneel on the floor. The distance between your knees should be the width of two fists. Place your forearms and the backs of your feet flat on the floor (**Fig. 7.13**).

Test

Can you touch your left and then your right knee with the tip of your nose, without tension or pain (**Fig. 7.13**)?

Exercise

Work toward the test objective until you feel the onset of tension. Remain in this position until the tension resolves.

▶ **Alternative test and exercise.** If the starting position in **Fig. 7.13** is unpleasant for your knees and the backs of your feet, a cushion and a rolled-up towel will help (**Fig. 7.14**). Make the cushion and the towel just thick enough so that your knees and the backs of your feet do not hurt in the starting position. Depending on the cause of the knee problems, the cushion may always be necessary. But if you exercise every day, the rolled towel at the back of your feet can usually be reduced from day to day, so that soon you will no longer need it.

Troubleshooting

If the tension does not diminish over the course of the exercise, the following tests and exercises should be used to detect and resolve possible mechanical impediments. If one of the following tests is positive, have your patient do the corresponding exercise and then repeat the stretching of the back muscles. If the tension has now resolved, you have found and solved the blockade.

If a costosternal syndrome is caused by habitual slouching, the irritated costochondral joints are stretched during thoracic extension. This can be temporarily felt as a painful pulling in this area, but it gradually disappears if the erect posture is maintained in spite of the pain.

If the intervertebral foramina in the thoracic spine are stenotic because of a herniated disk or because a vertebra in this area is twisted, extension of the thoracic spine can bring on or intensify symptoms in this area. In cases of a herniated disk, the symptoms decrease in the alternative supine position (**Fig. 7.11**). A twisted thoracic vertebra is often repositioned by the rotational mobility exercise (p. 90) or in the course of thoracic extension (**Fig. 7.9**) in combination with purely abdominal breathing (p. 47).

Irreversible limitations of thoracic extension due to Sheuermann disease, ankylosing spondylitis, or osteoporotic fractures, severely limit the thoracic extension that may be gained with the thoracic extension mobility exercises (**Fig. 7.9** and **Fig. 7.11**).

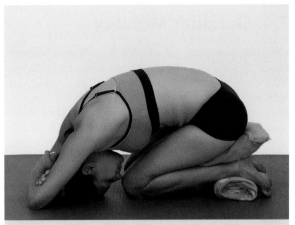

Fig. 7.13 Back muscle flexibility.

Fig. 7.14 Alternative test and exercise with a cushion and/or towel.

- Try the alternative exercise (**Fig. 7.14**)
- Repeat the exercise with less tension while simultaneously doing all the relaxation exercises (p. 39)
- Buttock muscle flexibility (p. 96)
- Posterior thigh flexibility (p. 101)
- Leg, back, and cranial nerve mobility (p. 98)
- Back muscle strength (p. 118)
- Anterior thigh flexibility (p. 113)

Before and After Comparison

How great is the distance between nose and knee at the closest point (**Fig. 7.15**)?

Differential Diagnosis

If a sacroiliac joint blockade is hindering the movement of the nose toward the knee, this is usually felt locally as pain in the sacroiliac region. In this case, it will be possible to move the nose closer to the knee after the sacroiliac joint has been repositioned manually or by means of the anterior thigh flexibility exercise (p. 113).

Biomechanics

The sitting posture of most people is slouched, with flexion of the lumbar, thoracic, and lower cervical spine. Only the middle and upper cervical spine is hyperextended in compensation, to allow the person to look straight ahead. In the long term, this hyperextension leads to a shortening of the neck muscles that may be felt as tension in the back muscle flexibility test. The same is true for all reflex (pp. 46 and 49) and parafunctional increases in neck muscle tone (pp. 39–49) due to a lack of relaxation.

In the lumbar and thoracic spine, no tension is usually felt during the back muscle flexibility test if the patient is below the age of 50, because the muscles in this area are typ-

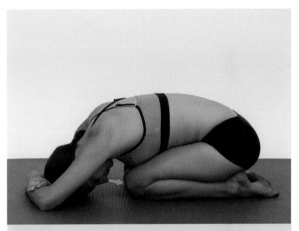

Fig. 7.15 The distance between the nose and the knee.

ically already overstretched as a result of slouching. In the less frequent cases where tension is felt in the lumbar and thoracic spine, it is usually due to tight back extensor muscles. Typical causes of this tightness are static sitting for long periods (pp. 50–53), long periods of standing with a hyperextended lumbar spine (p. 38), or reflex guarding caused by instability, twisted vertebrae, spinal stenosis, or pain in the area of the disks, vertebral joints, or spinal nerves.

A pleasant finish

Stretching the back extensor muscles using the back muscle flexibility exercise is usually considered particularly agreeable, because the stretching takes place in a position that unloads the spine and produces a slight traction in the cervical spine. The corrective and relaxing effect of this exercise makes it a pleasant finish to a fitness program.

7.4 Shoulder Mobility

▶ **Starting position.** Lie on your back. If you have not passed the chin tuck mobility and thoracic extension mobility tests (pp. 70 and 73), rest your head on a pillow. Your right arm should lie at your side. Slide your left hand under your back until the tip of your left middle finger touches your right elbow (**Fig. 7.16**, ①), and leave it there. Now move your right elbow away from your left middle finger, and place your right hand flat on your left shoulder so that the thumb touches your neck and the tips of your extended fingers touch the floor (**Fig. 7.17**).

Test

Can you press your left shoulder blade so flat on the floor that your left shoulder glides down past the palm (**Fig. 7.18**, ②) and towards the fingers (**Fig. 7.19**, ③) of your right hand, until it only contacts the fingers and no longer contacts the palm—all without tension or pain?

Exercise

Press your left shoulder blade toward the floor until you feel the onset of tension. Remain in this position until the tension resolves. Your right hand lets you feel the direction of movement and the progress you have made with the exercise. As soon as you have developed a sense for both these things, you will no longer need to monitor the exercise with the right hand and can let it lie loosely by your side (**Fig. 7.20**).

▶ **Alternative exercise.** Should the starting position with the hand under your back be painful, you should start with your hand under your buttocks instead (**Fig. 7.21**). With increasing mobility, you will be able to move your hand further and further upward toward the test position (**Fig. 7.16**) without pain.

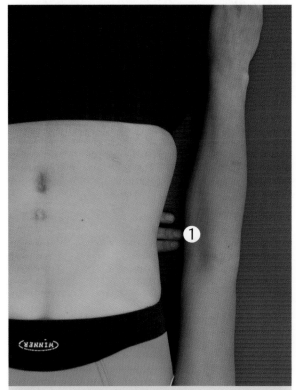

Fig. 7.16 Step 1: The fingertips of the left hand touch the right elbow.

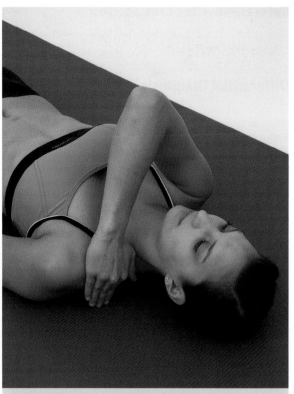

Fig. 7.17 Step 2: The right hand is placed on the left shoulder so that the thumb touches the neck and the fingertips touch the floor.

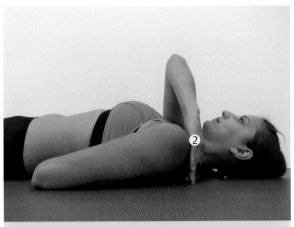

Fig. 7.18 The test has not been passed because the shoulder is only touching the palm of the hand—②.

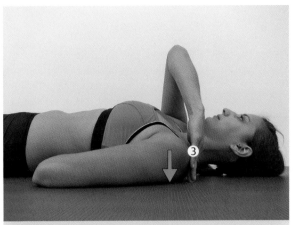

Fig. 7.19 The test has been passed, because the shoulder is pressed so flat on the floor that it now touches the fingers —③.

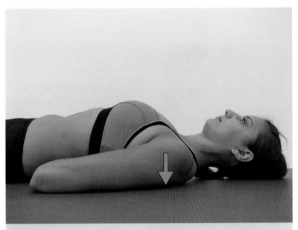

Fig. 7.20 The shoulder mobility exercise without using the right hand for measurement of progress.

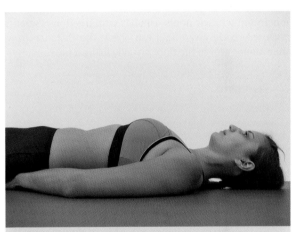

Fig. 7.21 The alternative starting position with the hand under the buttocks.

Troubleshooting

First retraction, then internal rotation

Patients with very limited shoulder mobility can hear an unpleasant crackling or rumbling in the shoulder joint when they place a hand under their back. They can usually avoid this by (1) first pulling the shoulder blade as far as possible toward the spine three times (adduction), and then (2) holding it there while placing their hand under their back. The unpleasant sounds disappear with increasing mobility.

If the shoulder tension does not lessen over the course of even the alternative exercise with the hand under the buttock (**Fig. 7.21**), the following tests and exercises should be used to detect and resolve possible mechanical impediments.

If one of the following tests is positive, have your patient do the corresponding exercise and then repeat the shoulder mobility exercise. If the tension has now resolved, you have found and solved the blockade.
- Repeat the exercise with less tension while simultaneously doing all the relaxation exercises (pp. 39–49)
- Rotational mobility (p. 90)
- Shoulder blade and triceps muscle strength (p. 120)
- Arm nerve mobility (p. 83)
- Thoracic extension mobility (p. 73)

If, because of limited mobility, the patient cannot place her right hand on her left shoulder during testing, the following alternative test is a possibility: Can the whole of the left upper arm, from the elbow to the axilla, be pressed onto the floor (**Fig. 7.22**)?

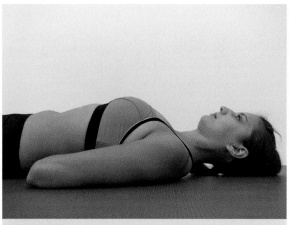

Fig. 7.22 The axilla is touching the floor.

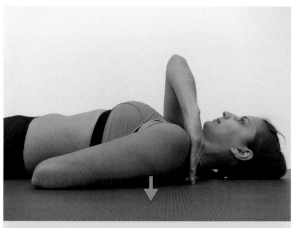

Fig. 7.23 A distance remains between the axilla and the floor.

Patients with a good sense of their body can feel how much contact their upper arm has with the floor. Patients with less body awareness can check the distance from their upper arm to the floor visually using a mirror.

Taut skin

This alternative test only works if the skin of the upper arm is taut. If the skin is not taut, the skin of the upper arm will touch the floor even with a protracted shoulder.

Before and After Comparison

In case the skin of the upper arm ist taut: How great is the distance between the floor and the upper arm at the axilla (**Fig. 7.23**)?

Otherwise: How far does the left hand (**Fig. 7.18**) have to move up away from the floor, so that the palm (**Fig. 7.18**, ②) will no longer contact the shoulder?

Differential Diagnosis

If the rotator cuff muscles are short or hypertonic, there is usually a feeling of tension in the lateral proximal half of the upper arm during the shoulder mobility exercise.

On the other hand, if the long tendon of the biceps is inflamed, the pain can usually be triggered by manual pressure between the major and minor tubercles (in the bicipital groove), as well as by tension of the biceps brachii in response to a contraction or stretch (**Fig. 7.24**).

Biomechanics

Tightness of the neck muscles that is only briefly improved by local treatment may compensate for another,

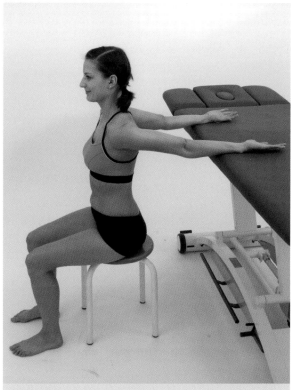

Fig. 7.24 Stretching the biceps brachii.

primary dysfunction. Other than costosternal breathing (p. 47) and a hypomobile brachial plexus (p. 83), this is often a limited internal rotation of the glenohumeral joint.

If the internal rotation of the glenohumeral joint is limited, the whole pectoral girdle must be protracted so that the hands can meet in the middle of the body. This shoulder protraction and the resulting kyphosis of the thoracic spine are important causes of neck tension and shoulder impingement (Betz et al 2005).

Conversely, the shoulder mobility exercise restores the ability to work with the hands at the body's center in a physiological posture. This, together with an increase in scapular retraction and improved circulation and elasticity in the rotator cuff tendon, may explain why symptoms of impingement decrease as progress is made with the shoulder mobility exercise.

7.5 Finger Flexor Flexibility

▶ **Starting position.** Stand an arm's length away from a corner of the room. Extend your left arm forward horizontally and turn it outward until the inside of your wrist, where you would feel your pulse, points upward and your elbow points downward. Then angle your wrist so that the fingers of your left hand point down, and touch the wall in front of you, while your left thumb and left shoulder are touching the wall to your left (**Fig. 7.25**).

Test

In this position, can you press the palm of your hand and your fingers flat against the wall in front of you (**Fig. 7.26**)?

Exercise

Push the palm of your hand toward the wall until you feel the onset of tension. Remain in this position until the tension resolves.

▶ **Alternative test and exercise.** Because your left shoulder is touching the wall, the starting position in the corner of a room prevents your torso from shifting to the left or right. In addition, this starting position permits a smooth transition to testing and practicing arm nerve mobility (p. 83).

If there is no suitable corner or if there are not enough corners for an exercise group, the test and the exercise for finger flexor flexibility can be done at a wall without a corner (**Fig. 7.27**).

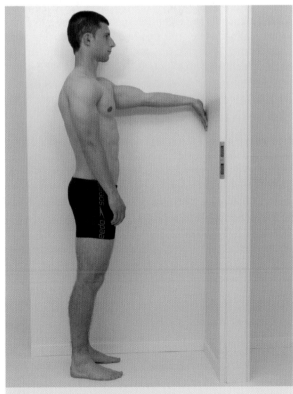

Fig. 7.25 With your arm horizontal ...

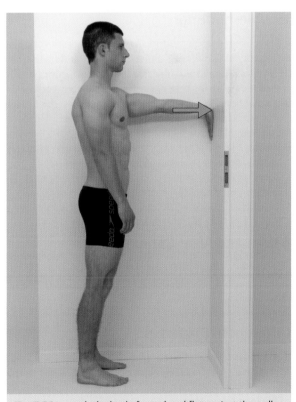

Fig. 7.26 ... push the heel of your hand flat against the wall.

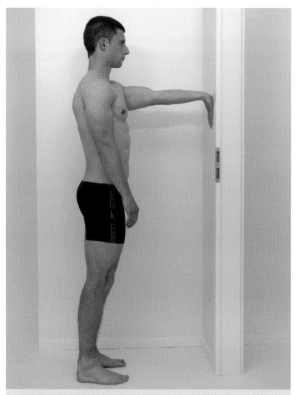

Fig. 7.27 Alternative test and exercise without a corner.

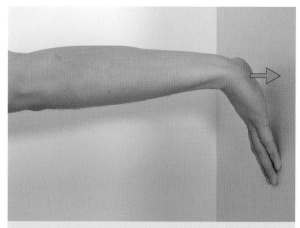

Fig. 7.28 The distance between the wall and the pisiform bone.

Troubleshooting

If the tension does not diminish over the course of the exercise, the following tests and exercises should be used to detect and resolve possible mechanical impediments. If one of the following tests is positive, have your patient do the corresponding exercise and then repeat the finger flexor stretch. If the tension has now resolved, you have found and solved the blockade.

- Repeat the exercise with less tension while simultaneously doing all the relaxation exercises (p. 39).
- Check the mobility of the lunate bone in the palmar direction, and if necessary mobilize it.
- Shoulder mobility (p. 78).

Before and After Comparison

How great is the distance between the wall and the hypothenar eminence at the level of the pisiform bone (**Fig. 7.28**)?

Differential Diagnosis

If your patient cannot reach the wall with the heel of her hypothenar eminence, the wrist extension may be limited by hypomobility at the wrist joints or deficient flexibility of the long finger flexors.

Insufficient flexibility of the long finger flexors is typically felt as a pull on the palmar side of the fingers, the palm, the wrist, or the lower arm, which fades with gentle stretching over the course of the exercise.

A blockade of the wrist joints, on the other hand, is usually experienced as pain or pressure centrally at the back of the wrist. The most common cause is a restricted palmar slide of the lunate bone. In cases of joint blockade, mobility and pain in the wrist will usually not improve with the finger flexor flexibility exercise. If the blockade, however, is resolved manually, the extension mobility in the wrist improves immediately. The exercise is then possible with considerably less pressure and more extension in the wrist, which leads to a more intense stretch of the finger flexor tendons.

Biomechanics

Free finger flexor flexibility relaxes the muscles of the forearm and as a result also the other muscles along the kinetic chain of the forearm–upper arm–shoulder–neck. Moreover, it permits an optimal support function of the arms, which takes stress off the spine, for instance, when rising from a supine to a sitting position.

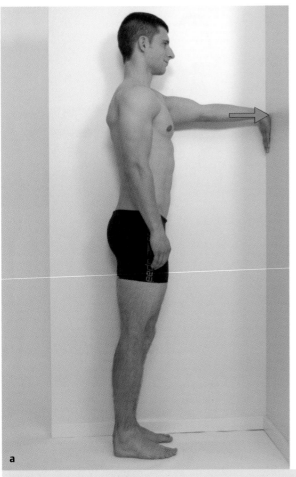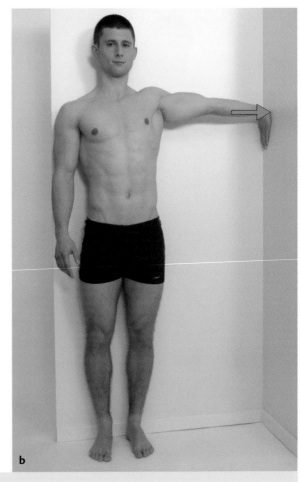

Fig. 7.29 Arm nerve mobility.

7.6 Arm Nerve Mobility

▶ **Starting position.** Stand in the same position as for the finger flexor flexibility test (**Figs. 7.26** or **7.29 a**).

Test

Can you keep the palm and the fingers of your left hand pressed flat against the wall, while you turn your feet and all the rest of your body so far to the right that both shoulders touch the wall (**Fig. 7.29 b**) without pain or additional tension in the fingers of your left hand, any other part of your left arm, or your left shoulder?

Exercise

Work toward the test objective until you feel the onset of tension. Remain in this position until the tension resolves.

Caution: Nerve irritation

You should proceed with particular care in this exercise since nerves are delicate and symptoms caused by over-exerting nerves often appear delayed.

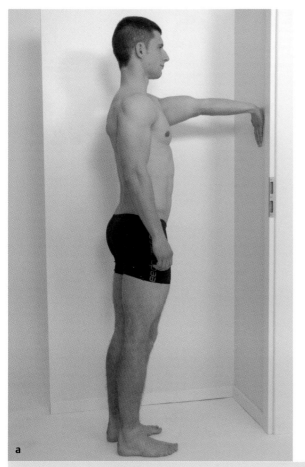
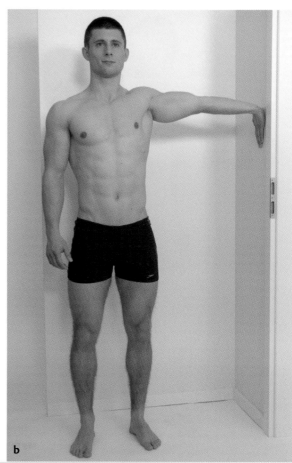

Fig. 7.30 Alternative exercise without a corner.

▶ **Alternative exercises.** If there is no appropriate corner or if there are not enough corners for an exercise group, the exercise can be done at a wall without a corner (**Fig. 7.30**).

The objective of the exercise is then to turn your feet and the entire rest of your body by a quarter turn to the right (**Fig. 7.30 b**) without pain or additional tension in the fingers of your left hand, any other part of your left arm, or your left shoulder.

If the neurodynamics of the brachial plexus are limited by a disk protrusion or degenerative changes of the cervical vertebrae, relaxation during the exercise often only occurs if the head is bent forward (**Fig. 7.31**) or if the patient is lying down with a thick pillow for sufficient cervical spine flexion (**Fig. 7.32**).

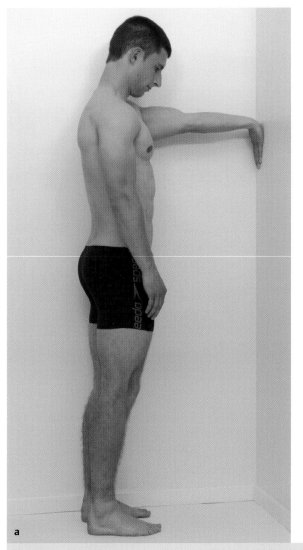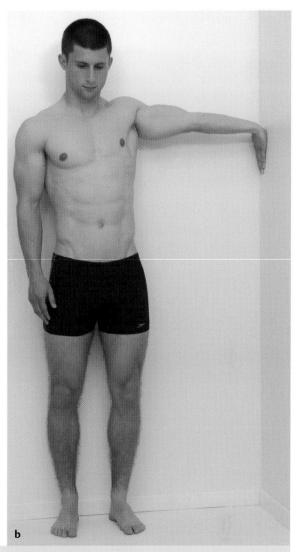

Fig. 7.31 Practicing arm nerve mobility, standing with the head bent forward.

Nerve stretch exercises

Exercises must be simple so that the patient can perform them herself. For this reason, a simple, static form of nerve mobilization was selected for the arm nerve mobility exercises demonstrated up to this point. In these exercises, the nerves are stretched until tension is felt. This position is held until the feeling of tension generated in this manner decreases perceptibly.

Nerve glide exercises

Patients with sufficient body awareness can also learn the dynamic form of nerve mobilization under the direction of their physical therapists. This form is also known as gliding exercises or sliders. In this exercise, the nerve is put under tension at one end and simultaneously given slack at the other end in continuous alternation (**Figs. 7.33** and **7.34**). As a result, the nerve glides back and forth, like a piece of dental floss between the teeth, along the adjacent tissues without itself being tensed. These gliding exercises are particularly gentle for nerves and are therefore recommended for acutely irritated and very sensitive nerves.

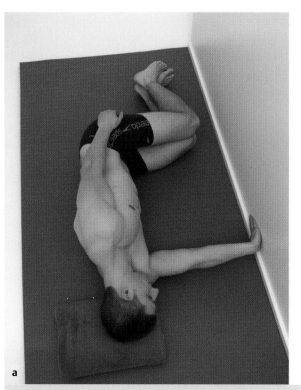
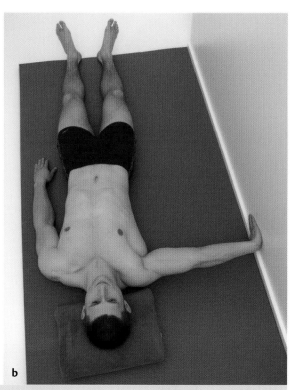

a

b

Fig. 7.32 Performing the arm nerve mobility exercise supine with a thick pillow.

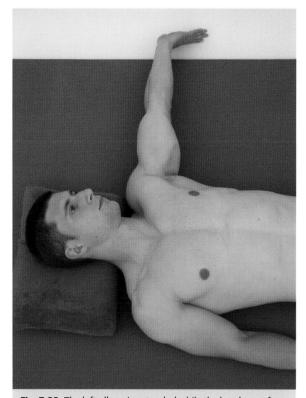
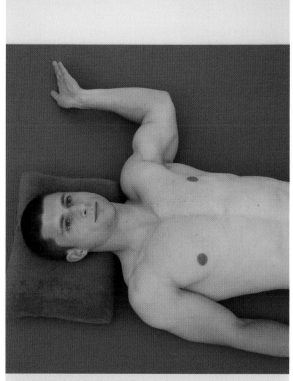

Fig. 7.33 The left elbow is extended while the head turns from its middle position toward the left elbow.

Fig. 7.34 The left elbow is flexed while the head returns to its middle position.

Troubleshooting

If the tension does not diminish over the course of the exercise, the following tests and exercises should be used to detect and resolve possible mechanical impediments. If one of the following tests is positive, have your patient do the corresponding exercise and then repeat the arm nerve mobility exercise. If the tension has diminished, you have found and eliminated the mechanical impediment.

- Repeat the exercise with less tension while simultaneously doing all the relaxation exercises (pp. 39–49)
- Thoracic extension mobility (p. 73)
- Rotational mobility (p. 90)
- Alternative exercises in this section (**Figs. 7.31**, **7.32**, **7.33**, **7.34**)
- Mobilization of the first rib (see **Fig. 11.1**)

Before and After Comparison

The test is passed if the patient can turn so far to the right, without tension, that both shoulders touch the wall (**Fig. 7.35**). If the test is not passed, measure the distance remaining between the medial edge of the right scapula and the wall (**Fig. 7.36**). If a patient cannot press the hypothenar eminence all the way to the wall, the distance between the pisiform bone and the wall is added (see **Fig. 7.28**).

Distance 1 + Distance 2

If the distance between the edge of the scapula and the wall is 4 cm in the test, and there is an additional distance of 1 cm between the pisiform bone and the wall, a total of 5 cm is recorded.

In the alternative exercise without a corner (see **Fig. 7.30**), the distance between the edge of the scapula and the wall cannot be measured. The before and after comparison of the upper body rotation must then be made by means of a less precise evaluation, in degrees or hours on an imaginary clock face.

Differential Diagnosis

A decrease in tension in the test position (**Fig. 7.37**) in response to manual cervical spine traction applied by the therapist (**Fig. 7.38**) indicates a nerve impingement at the disk or the intervertebral foramen. In this case, it is worthwhile seeing whether the patient's symptoms and neurodynamics can be more effectively improved using one of the alternative exercises in **Figs. 7.31**, **7.32**, **7.33**, **7.34**.

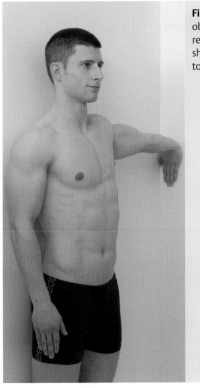

Fig. 7.35 The test objective has been reached: Both shoulders are touching the wall.

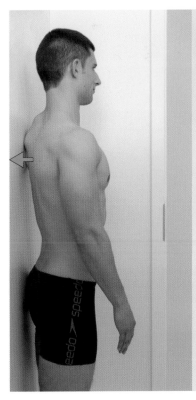

Fig. 7.36 The test has not been passed: A space remains between the medial edge of the right scapula and the wall.

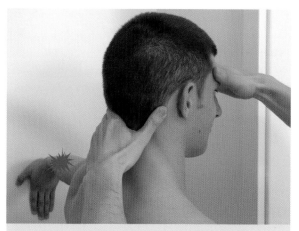

Fig. 7.37 Tension in the test position without traction.

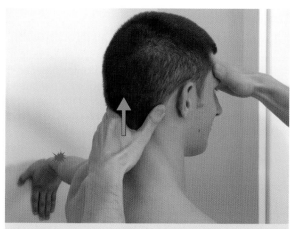

Fig. 7.38 Tension decreased by traction of the cervical spine.

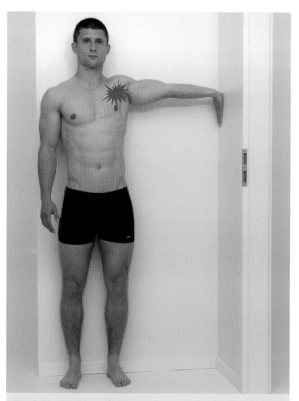

Fig. 7.39 Tension in the test position.

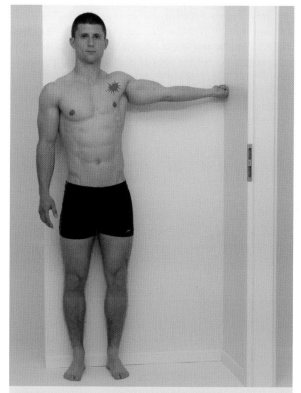

Fig. 7.40 Tension decreased by making a fist.

If you want to be sure that the test-related symptoms in a certain region really come from neural tension, you can relax the nerve by moving a part of the body that is as far removed as possible and connected to the symptomatic region only by nerves, and not by muscles, bones, or joint structures.

Neural versus local

Tension in the pectoralis minor muscle is felt in the position shown in **Fig. 7.39** and can be dissipated by making a fist with the ipsilateral hand (**Fig. 7.40**). This is a strong indication of a neurodynamic cause because the nerves are the only mechanical connection between the fingers and the chest. Analogously, a neurodynamically based symptom in the hand can be intensified by contralateral lateral flexion of the cervical spine.

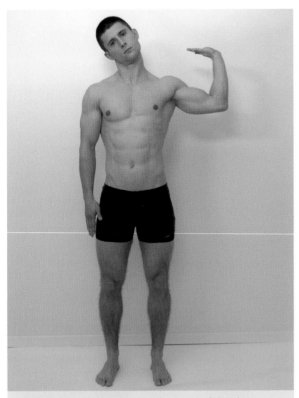

Fig. 7.41 Neurodynamic test and exercise of the ulnar nerve.

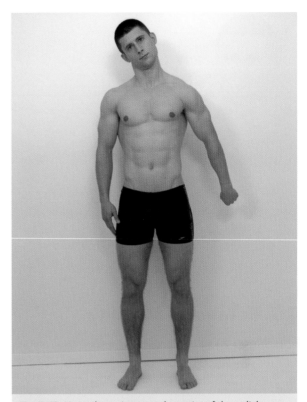

Fig. 7.42 Neurodynamic test and exercise of the radial nerve.

The arm nerve mobility exercises shown up to now mobilize all parts of the brachial plexus, with special emphasis on the median nerve component, and are in most cases sufficient for treating limited arm nerve mobility.

The more rarely affected plexus portions of the ulnar or radial nerve may be emphasized as follows:

- Ulnar nerve (**Fig. 7.41**)
  - Cervical spine: contralateral lateral flexion
  - Shoulder: abduction, depression, and external rotation
  - Elbow: flexion
  - Lower arm: pronation
  - Wrist: extension
  - Fingers: maximal stretching

- Radial nerve (**Fig. 7.42**)
  - Cervical spine: contralateral lateral flexion
  - Shoulder: depression, internal rotation, and as much abduction as the depressed shoulder allows
  - Elbow: extension
  - Lower arm: pronation
  - Wrist: flexion and ulnar deviation
  - Fingers: fist

Biomechanics

Neurodynamics

Free arm nerve mobility prevents neurodynamically induced pain and tension in the head, face, cervical spine, and arm.

Muscle guarding often serves to keep hypomobile nerves slack. This type of muscle tension (**Fig. 7.43**) can only be resolved long term by restoring free nerve mobility.

In the case of the brachial plexus, this particularly affects the shoulder elevators (levator scapulae, the descending part of trapezius, and scalenus) and the shoulder protractors (pectoralis major and minor). If the nerve roots of the median nerve are under tension, the flexors of the elbow, hand, and fingers are also affected. In the case of the ulnar nerve, these are the triceps brachii and the wrist—and finger—flexors, and in the case of the radial nerve, the triceps brachii and the wrist—and finger—extensors.

If the hypertonicity of these muscles can only be decreased short term with other therapeutic methods, limited nerve mobility may be the underlying cause. If so, only identifying and mobilizing the respective nerve will provide a lasting solution.

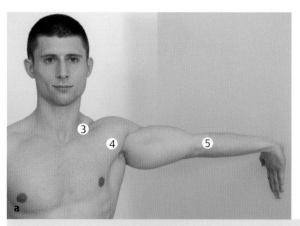 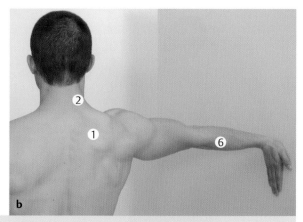

Fig. 7.43 Typical areas of muscle hypertonicity due to muscle guarding of hypomobile nerves: Levator scapulae ①, upper trapezius ②, scalene muscles ③, pectoralis major and minor ④, wrist and finger flexors ⑤, and hand and finger extensors ⑥.

7.7 Rotational Mobility

▸ **Starting position.** Lie on your right side. Place your left hand under your head so that your fingers touch the posterior edge of your right ear. If you have not passed the chin tuck mobility (p. 70) and thoracic extension mobility (p. 73) tests, you should place a pillow between your head and your left hand. Now grasp the middle of the back of your left knee with the tips of your right-hand fingers, and pull your left leg toward the floor until your right elbow touches the floor (**Fig. 7.44**, ①).

Test

Can you hold your left knee and your right elbow (**Fig. 7.44**, ①) in this position (without tension or pain) while at the same time bringing your left elbow backward until your left arm touches the floor (**Fig. 7.44**, ②)?

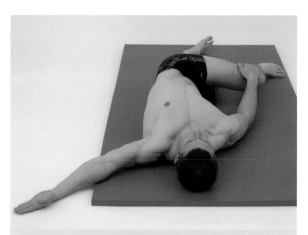

Fig. 7.44 Rotational mobility test.

Exercise

Extend your left elbow and let your arm sink toward the floor until you feel the onset of tension (**Fig. 7.45**). Remain in this position until the tension resolves. When you no longer feel tension in this position, you can try to see whether you feel more tension if you slide your left arm a little further upward or downward along the floor.

Fig. 7.45 Rotational mobility exercise.

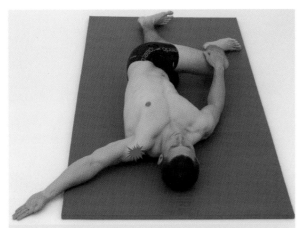

Fig. 7.46 If there is pain on the top of the shoulder …

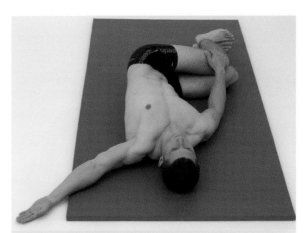

Fig. 7.48 Alternative exercise with the knees lying on top of each other.

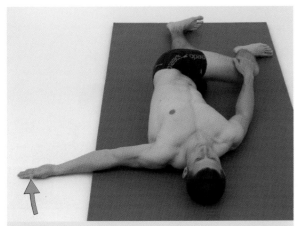

Fig. 7.47 … let the arm slide down along the floor until the pain has gone.

▶ **Alternative exercises.** If your shoulder joint is maligned, various tendons in the left shoulder joint can be pinched during the rotational mobility exercise. This pinching is called impingement and typically causes pain on the top of the shoulder, at the point where shoulder pads in jackets, pullovers, or blouses are located (**Fig. 7.46**). This impingement is counterproductive because it adds to the irritation of the impinged tendon. So if there is pain, slide your left arm downward along the floor (**Fig. 7.47**) until the pain disappears.

If the exercise causes pain in the spine or around your sacrum, you should concentrate on letting each individual thoracic vertebra and each rib go along with the rotation, and letting the left arm be pulled down by gravity. If this does not eliminate the symptoms, see whether laying your knees on top of each other helps (**Fig. 7.48**).

Troubleshooting

The typical imbalance within the spinal rotation movement chain is that the thoracic spine becomes hypomobile while the lower lumbar spine, sacroiliac joints, and midcervical spine become hypermobile and symptomatic. In this case, symptoms arising in the sacroiliac joint or lumbar spine during the exercise often disappear immediately once the patient releases subconscious en-bloc tensions in the thorax. She can achieve this by consciously allowing each individual thoracic vertebra and each rib to go along with the rotation, and by allowing her left arm to follow the pull of gravity.

If the tension in the shoulder–arm region still does not diminish over the course of the exercise, the following tests and exercises should be used to detect and resolve possible mechanical impediments. If one of the following tests is positive, have your patient do the corresponding exercise and then repeat the rotational mobility exercise. If the tension has now resolved, you have found and solved the blockade.
- Repeat the exercise with less tension while simultaneously doing all the relaxation exercises (p. 39)
- Shoulder mobility (p. 78)
- Shoulder blade and triceps muscle strength (p. 120)
- Manual release of the pectoralis minor muscle (see **Fig. 11.3**)
- Manual mobilization of the glenohumeral joint (see **Fig. 11.2**)

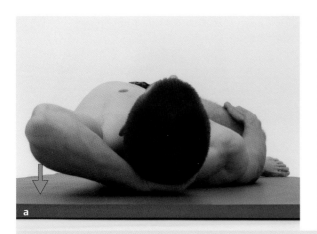

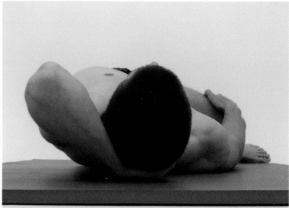

Fig. 7.49 A short distance between the floor and the forearm (**a**). A greater distance between the floor and the forearm (**b**).

Before and After Comparison

How great is the distance between the floor and the point on the left forearm that would touch the floor first (**Fig. 7.49 a**)?

A large distance between forearm and floor (**Fig. 7.49 b**) makes it difficult to decide which point this might be. In this case, you may identify the point immediately before the test by having the patient turn her whole body to the left until her left forearm touches the floor (**Fig. 7.50**). The point on the left forearm that touches the floor first is the point from which the distance to the floor will be measured in the subsequent test.

Differential Diagnosis

The rotational mobility exercise (**Fig. 7.45**) mobilizes chiefly the muscles and fasciae of the left hip abductors, spine, thorax, and left arm. When symptoms appear in the left arm during this exercise, one option to differentiate whether they are triggered by neurodynamic or myofascial tension are the arm nerve mobility tests (p. 83). An increase in symptoms during these tests is indicative of neurodynamic dysfunction. If, however, the arm nerve mobility tests are passed without increasing the symptoms, hypomobility of the brachial plexus as a cause of the symptoms can be ruled out.

Biomechanics

The rotational mobility exercise is an unspecific mobilization technique that affects a multitude of joints and tissues from the attachments of the iliotibial tract at the tibia and the patellofemoral joint, all the way up to the cervical spine. This exercise mobilizes the brachial plexus, the musculoskeletal components, and the viscera, as well as the interfaces between these systems, for example the mobility between the thorax and lungs in the pleural

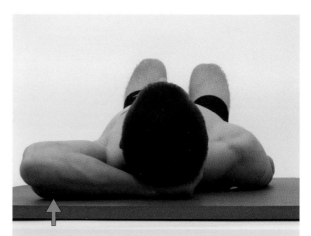

Fig. 7.50 This point on the forearm touched the floor first.

space. Another relevant interface is the passage of the brachial plexus and the blood vessels of the arm under the pectoralis minor muscle. Increased tension in the pectoralis minor and major muscles compresses the nerves and blood vessels that pass underneath, and also impedes the normal function of the shoulder and the spine.

Compression of the arm nerves and blood vessels due to tight chest muscles may cause tingling in the hand and forearm if the tension of the tight muscle is raised even further by means of a contraction or a stretch, for example when sleeping with one arm over the head or while practicing the rotational mobility exercise (**Fig. 7.45**). If the tingling becomes unpleasant during the exercise, the patient should pause briefly until it is gone and then resume the exercise. Once the pectoral muscle relaxes during the exercise, the load on the underlying nerves and blood vessels immediately eases. When the objective of the test is achieved through faithful practice (see **Fig. 7.44**), the tingling should no longer occur during daily activities or the exercise.

> **Paresthesias**
>
> Paresthesias in the hand and arm that occur during exercising are not a contraindication to the exercise; on the contrary, they indicate that the rotational mobility exercise may serve to reduce the paresthesias in the long run.

Finally, a relaxation of the pectoral muscle often causes twisted vertebrae between C7 and T2 to realign. This may be because a tense pectoral muscle protracts the shoulder blade, resulting in hypertonicity of the antagonists, namely the rhomboid muscles and the transverse portion of the trapezius muscle. If tense, their attachment to the spinous processes of C7–T4 and C7–T3 may cause a twisting of the respective vertebrae, that resolves with relaxation of the pectoral muscle.

7.8 Lifting Technique

▶ **Starting position.** Stand in front of a bottle containing 1.5 L of water that is placed before you on the floor.

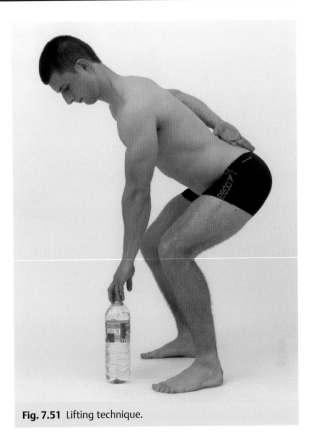

Fig. 7.51 Lifting technique.

Test

Can you lift the bottle (without tension or pain) with a stabilized neutral spinal curvature (p. 23) without raising your heels from the floor (**Fig. 7.51**)?

Exercise

Work toward the test objective until you feel the first resistance. Remain in this position until the resistance resolves.

▶ **Alternative exercise.** It makes sense to practice the right lifting technique whenever something must be lifted during your daily activities. Until you pass the test, however, you should place things that you regularly lift high enough that you can pick them up with a stabilized neutral spinal curvature (p. 23). For instance, you could set the bottle crate that you frequently have to lift on top of another bottle crate.

Troubleshooting

If the tension does not diminish over the course of the exercise, the following tests and exercises should be used to detect and resolve possible mechanical impediments. If one of the following tests is positive, have your patient do the corresponding exercise and then repeat the lifting technique. If it is now easier, you have found and solved the blockade.

If your patient cannot reach the bottle with a stabilized spine, refer to the "Before and After Comparison" for this section and note how much the distance between hand and bottle is decreased by the following exercises:
- Posterior thigh flexibility (p. 101)
- Hip flexion mobility (p. 95)
- Buttock muscle flexibility (p. 96)
- Anterior thigh flexibility (p. 113)
- Leg, back, and cranial nerve mobility (p. 98)

If the patient pronates her subtalar joint while reaching for the bottle, you should teach her not to use this compensatory movement but to actively maintain a stabilized arch during this movement. If the patient is not able to do this or raises her heel while trying to reach the bottle, you should examine the mobility of her talocrural joint. In cases of a restriction, the movement sequence can be normalized by means of manual mobilization of the talocrural joint (p. 145).

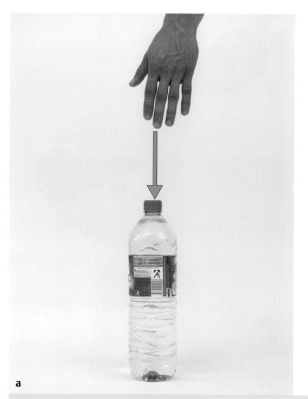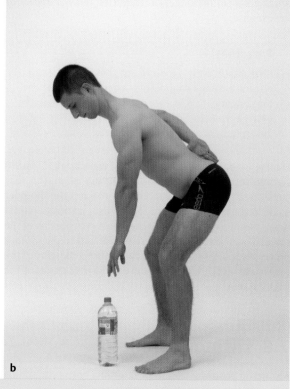

Fig. 7.52 The distance between the hand and the bottle.

Before and After Comparison

How great is the distance between the hand and the bottle (**Fig. 7.52**)?

Differential Diagnosis

If the bottle cannot be reached without raising the heels, the cause can lie either in the muscles or in the joints. If talocrural dorsiflexion is restricted, the patient will feel pressure at the anterior aspect of the joint. If it is primarily the flexibility of the soleus muscle that is restricted, tension will be felt in this muscle or in the Achilles tendon. However, this is rare, occurring only with marked adhesion or shortness of the soleus muscle.

In both cases, the patient will tend to compensate for the lack of dorsiflexion by compensatory pronation.

Talocrural hypomobility

Often a muscular restriction can only be felt after a primary joint hypomobility has been resolved.

Biomechanics

A correct lifting technique prevents disk injuries by maintaining the lordosis of the lumbar spine and lifting with the legs. For this reason, the technique requires and trains free hip flexion mobility (p. 95). In addition to avoiding acute back injuries, the technique also prevents degenerative wear that arises from the typical imbalance between hypomobile hips and a hypermobile lumbar spine. In order to prevent this imbalance, the correct lifting technique may also be applied to lifting light objects that pose no threat of acute injury. When applied in this way, the lifting technique serves as a quick and practical lumbar stabilization and hip flexion exercise, which can be easily integrated into daily activities and compensates somewhat for the slouched posture of a predominantly sedentary lifestyle.

7.9 Hip Flexion Mobility

▶ **Starting position.** Sit on a stool or chair of adequate height (p. 28), facing the wall. Leave a forearm's length between your knees (**Fig. 7.53**) and a distance the width of two fists between your knees and the wall (**Fig. 7.54**). Then slide forward or backward on your seat until your shins are vertical.

Now place your fist against your voice box and slide your chin backward on your fist until you feel a slight tension in your neck (p. 72) and hold this position while you lean forward with a stabilized neutral spinal curvature (p. 23).

Test

Can you lean forward with a stabilized neutral spinal curvature (p. 23)—in other words while keeping your lower back arched—until your head touches the wall (**Fig. 7.55**), without tension or pain?

Exercise

Work toward the test objective until you feel the first resistance. Remain in this position until the resistance resolves.

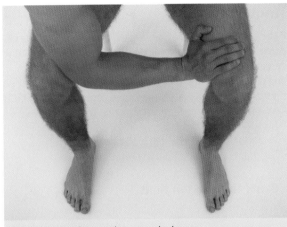

Fig. 7.53 The distance between the knees.

▶ **Alternative exercise.** During the exercise, you should keep your lower back arched to the extent described under neutral spinal curvature (p. 12). Balance your upper body (p. 25) and see if you can arch your lower back in this position. If not, raise the height of your seat until you can, and leave it at that height for both everyday purposes and for exercising hip flexor mobility. If the height of your chair is not adjustable, raise the seat height with a cushion or choose a higher chair.

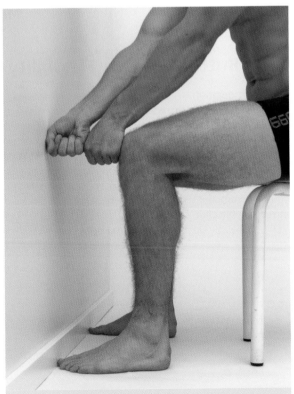

Fig. 7.54 The distance between the knees and the wall.

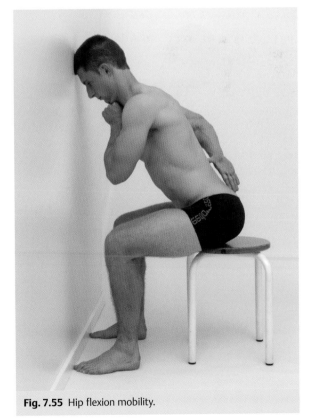

Fig. 7.55 Hip flexion mobility.

Troubleshooting

If the mobility does not improve over the course of the exercise, the following tests and exercises should be used to detect and resolve possible mechanical impediments. If one of the following tests is positive, have your patient do the corresponding exercise and then repeat the test. If it is now easier, you have found and solved the blockade.

- Buttock muscle flexibility (p. 96)
- Posterior thigh flexibility (p. 101)
- Leg, back, and cranial nerve mobility (p. 98)

Pants that are too tight

If your patient's pants are too tight for the seated exercises (see "Differential Diagnosis" for this section), the immediate solution is for your patient to leave them unbuttoned, unzipped, or to take them off. The next step is to buy wider pants that do not restrict hip flexion mobility.

Before and After Comparison

At the narrowest point, how great is the distance between the patient's head and the wall (**Fig. 7.56**)?

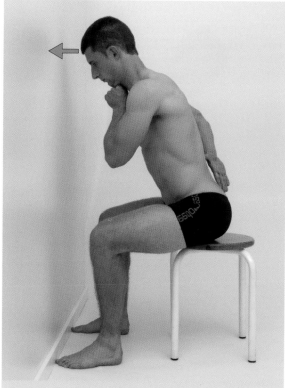

Fig. 7.56 The distance between the head and the wall.

Differential Diagnosis

An end range hip flexion of a hypomobile hip joint typically elicits a feeling of impingement in the middle of the groin. If a groin pain increases with coughing or if a bulge is visible in the groin area, an inguinal hernia needs to be ruled out.

Depending on whether the restriction is muscular or neurodynamic in origin, hip flexion mobility will be improved in proportion to the practice of hip flexion mobility (p. 95), buttock muscle flexibility (p. 96), posterior thigh flexibility (p. 101), or leg, back, or cranial nerve mobility (p. 98) exercises.

Quite often pants that are too tight are the primary impediment to free hip flexor mobility. If this kind of "textile contracture" is present, hip flexion is noticeably easier with a loosened belt, pants' button, or zipper.

Biomechanics

Neutral spinal curvature (see **Fig. 3.4**, p. 12) is only possible with free hip flexion mobility, which allows a neutral alignment of the pelvis while sitting, lifting, or bending forward. If hip flexion mobility is restricted, the adjacent joints of the flexion mobility chain (the sacroiliac joint and L5–S1 joints) must compensate by proportionate hypermobility. Consequently, a hip flexion deficit promotes instability of the sacroiliac joint and wear of the disk between L5 and S1.

7.10 Buttock Muscle Flexibility

▶ **Starting position.** Sit on a chair or stool of adequate height (p. 28), facing the wall, and touch the wall with the toes of your right foot and your right knee. Place your left foot on your right thigh so that your left knee and the toenails of your left foot also touch the wall. Let your left knee fall loosely outward. Maintain your lumbar spine in natural lordosis with 75% extension (p. 12). Place your fist on your sternum and slide your chin backward on your fist into a "double chin" position (p. 72, see **Fig. 7.5**).

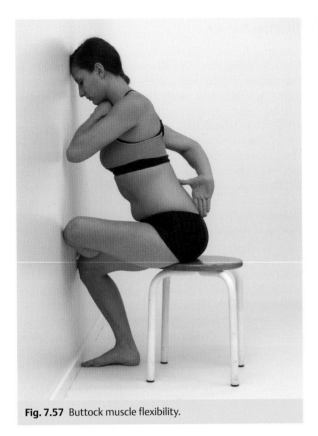

Fig. 7.57 Buttock muscle flexibility.

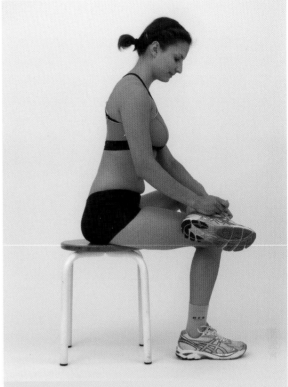

Fig. 7.58 Buttock muscle flexibility exercise when taking the shoes off.

Exercise

Work toward the test objective until you feel the first resistance. Remain in this position until the resistance resolves.

▶ **Alternative exercise**

• Seated

Buttock muscle flexibility can also be practiced without a wall. For instance, integrate the buttock muscle flexibility exercise into everyday activity by holding the stretched position described above while putting on and taking off your shoes and socks (**Fig. 7.58**). If you cannot stabilize (p. 23) the neutral spinal curvature (p. 12) and let your back become rounded, you should raise the height of your seat until you can keep your lower back arched. If the height of your chair is not adjustable, you can raise the seat height with a cushion or choose a higher chair.

• On your hands and knees

To stretch your left buttock muscle, place the right side of your groin on your left heel. Then arch your lower back and shift your hips to the left without letting the right side of your groin lose contact with your left heel. Continue until you feel the onset of tension in your left buttock muscle (**Fig. 7.59**). Hold this position until the tension disappears.

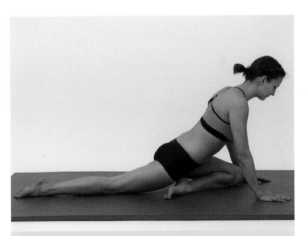

Fig. 7.59 Buttock muscle flexibility exercise on the hands and knees.

Troubleshooting

If the tension does not diminish over the course of the exercise, the following tests and exercises should be used to detect and resolve possible mechanical impediments. If one of the following tests is positive, have your patient do the corresponding exercise and then repeat the buttock muscle flexibility exercise. If the tension has now resolved, you have found and solved the blockade.

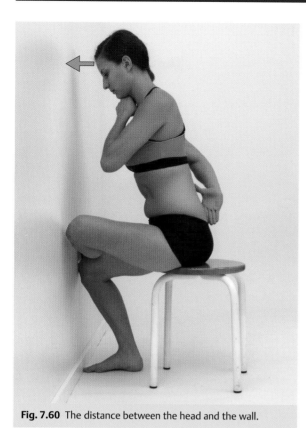

Fig. 7.60 The distance between the head and the wall.

- Repeat the exercise with less tension while simultaneously doing all the relaxation exercises (p. 39)
- Posterior thigh flexibility (p. 101)
- Leg, back, and cranial nerve mobility (p. 98)
- Hip flexion mobility (p. 95)
- Hip extension mobility (p. 109)
- Anterior thigh flexibility (p. 113)

Before and After Comparison

At the narrowest point, how great is the distance between the patient's head and the wall (**Fig. 7.60**)?

Differential Diagnosis

An impingement in the groin that comes on during stretching of the buttock muscles may be caused by hip arthritis, anterior migration of the femoral head, or malalignment of the sacroiliac joint. If the cause is anterior migration of the femoral head, the feeling of impingement in the groin decreases after doing the alternative exercise on the hands and knees (**Fig. 7.59**), the hip extension mobility exercise (p. 109), or the anterior thigh flexibility exercise (p. 113).

Biomechanics

Like good hamstring flexibility, complete flexibility of the buttocks prevents the development of hypermobility in the sacroiliac joint and the L5–S1 segment as adjacent joints during kinetic chain flexion. An improvement in buttock muscle flexibility thus decreases the load on the L5–S1 disk, where 58% of lumbar disk herniations are found, compared with only 36% for the L4–L5 and 5% for the L3–L4 disks (Schäfer 2005). Complete buttock muscle flexibility facilitates a neutral spinal curvature (p. 12), particularly when the hip is flexed and externally rotated, for instance when sitting cross-legged or when putting on or taking off the shoes and socks while sitting on a chair with one leg crossed over the other.

Moreover, complete buttock muscle flexibility makes normal functioning of the sciatic nerve possible, as the nerve passes under and in some individuals even through the piriformis muscle. Because of this close relationship, elevated tension in the piriformis muscle can irritate the sciatic nerve, compress it, and hamper its neurodynamics (Fishman et al 2004).

> **Piriformis muscle**
>
> The piriformis muscle is stretched when the hip is flexed and adducted. Once the hip is flexed, as in the buttock muscle flexibility exercise, it is also stretched by external rotation of the hip, since beyond 60° flexion the muscle changes from being an external to an internal rotator of the hip (Snijders et al 2006).

7.11 Leg, Back, and Cranial Nerve Mobility

▶ **Starting position.** Sit on the front edge of a chair or stool of adequate height (p. 28), facing the wall. Your toes should be a foot's length away from the wall, and your shins should be vertical. Place your left foot with the heel on the floor and the ball of your foot against the wall, as in stepping on the clutch of a car (**Fig. 7.61**, ①).

Test

Can you bend forward from this position (slowly and carefully, since the nerves are sensitive) until your hands are flat on the floor (without tension or pain), and can you see the underside of your chair (**Fig. 7.61**, ②)?

This assumes that the underside of your chair is flat. If the chair curves down at the front end, imagine you can see through the curve.

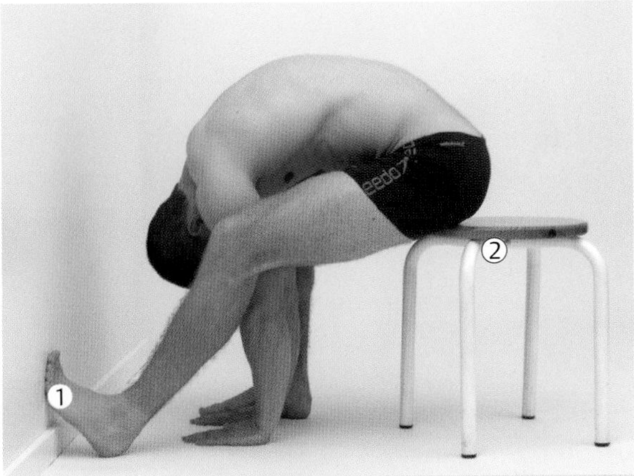

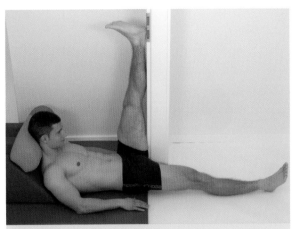

Fig. 7.61 Leg, back, and cranial nerve mobility.

Fig. 7.62 Leg, back, and cranial nerve mobility exercise in the supine position.

Exercise

Work toward the test objective until you feel the onset of tension. Remain in this position until the tension resolves.

▶ **Alternative exercise.** Practicing the leg, back, and cranial nerve mobility exercise should not cause any discomfort in the lumbar spine. If symptoms do arise in the lumbar spine when the exercise is done in a seated position (**Fig. 7.61**), see whether they can be avoided using an alternative exercise in the supine position. The exercise functions similarly to the posterior thigh flexibility exercise (p. 101), except that the cervical and thoracic spine must be flexed as far as comfortably possible with the help of cushions (**Fig. 7.62**).

If your therapist concludes that the release of tension during the alternative exercise in the supine position (**Fig. 7.62**) is impeded by pinching of the sciatic nerve roots on one side of the lumbar spine, the impingement may be reduced by bending the lumbar spine to the opposite side (**Fig. 7.63**).

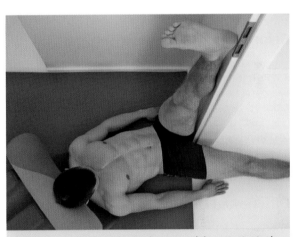

Fig. 7.63 Leg, back, and cranial nerve mobility exercise in the supine position with side bending.

Caution: Herniated disks

In cases of a preexisting lumbar disk injury, it is best to wait at least an hour after getting up before doing the exercise (**Fig. 7.61**), so that the pressure and stiffness of the disk, and its susceptibility to injury, decreases. If pain still arises in the lumbar spine during exercise, check whether the exercises in a supine position (see **Figs. 7.62** and **7.63**) will provide a pain-free alternative.

Troubleshooting

If the tension does not diminish over the course of the exercise, the following tests and exercises should be used to detect and resolve possible mechanical impediments. If one of the following tests is positive, have your patient do the corresponding exercise and then repeat the leg, back, and cranial nerve flexibility exercise. If the tension has now resolved, you have found and solved the blockade.

- Repeat the exercise with less tension while simultaneously doing all the relaxation exercises (p. 39)
- Alternative exercises in the supine position (**Figs. 7.62** and **7.63**)
- Posterior thigh flexibility (p. 101)
- Buttock muscle flexibility (p. 96)
- Anterior thigh flexibility (p. 113)
- Calf flexibility (p. 103)
- Back muscle strength (p. 118)

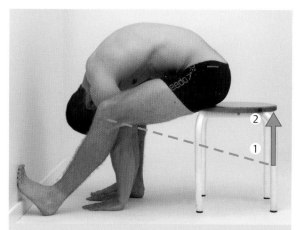

Fig. 7.64 The blue arrow marks the length of the section of the stool's back leg that the patient does not see.

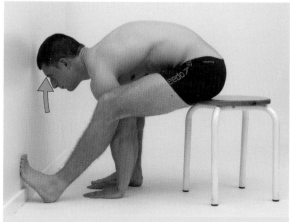

Fig. 7.65 Differentiation through cervical spine extension.

Before and After Comparison

Slide the index finger of one hand up along the back leg of a stool until the index finger disappears from the patient's view (the broken line in **Fig. 7.64**). How great is the distance between the underside of the index finger (**Fig. 7.64**, ①) and the underside of the stool (**Fig. 7.64**, ②)? In other words, how long is the section of the stool's back leg that the patient cannot see (**Fig. 7.64**, blue arrow)?

Differential Diagnosis

In order to determine whether the symptoms that arise during practice of the leg, back, and cranial nerve mobility exercise are neurodynamic in origin, the neural tension should be released at a spot that has no muscle or joint connection with the symptomatic area.

For instance, if tension is felt in the dorsal thigh during the exercise, only the cervical spine should be extended (**Fig. 7.65**). If cervical spine extension reduces this tension, the corresponding component of the tension was neurodynamic in origin. If it does not, the tension was myofascial in origin.

On the other hand, if the exercise causes tension in the head or spinal region, the neural tension can be decreased for purposes of differentiation by retracting the foot that is against the wall and placing it next to the other foot (**Fig. 7.66**). If the tension decreases as a result, the corresponding component of the tension was neurodynamic in origin. If the tension persists, it is an indication of myofascial origin.

The seated exercise (**Fig. 7.61**) may cause a sense of pressure in the head, which is usually caused by an elevation of craniofacial blood pressure in this position. If this is the

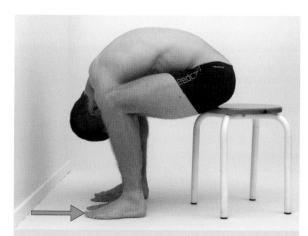

Fig. 7.66 Differentiation by retracting the foot.

case, the pressure would be the same during the back muscle flexibility exercise (p. 76), but significantly less in the alternative leg, back, and cranial nerve mobility exercise in the supine position (**Fig. 7.62**).

Biomechanics

- Consequences of restricted neurodynamics
  The dura mater is mechanically connected to the sacrum, the cranial bones, the cranial and spinal nerves, and, through the dural ligaments, to the vertebral bodies and the foramen magnum. Via these connections, tension in the dura is transmitted to the entire spine and the cranial and spinal nerves, and may cause dysfunction and pain. Typical examples of this are frontal or parietal headaches that respond to the differential testing of leg, back, and cranial nerve mobility, dull diffuse pain in the thoracic spine area, a dysfunction in the co-

ordination of the eyes (a positive eye muscle coordination test, p. 65), and twisted vertebrae.

Furthermore, a restriction of dural dynamics leads to reflex hypertonicity of the neck extensors. Lasting relaxation of the neck extensors is then only possible by restoration of free dural mobility.

> **Dura mater**
>
> A release of dural tension usually produces an immediate improvement in all the findings mentioned.

- Neurodynamics in response to variations in disk height. When the disk height increases, the spine expands in a vertical direction, causing the tension of the dura and the sciatic nerve to increase accordingly. The reverse happens when the disk height decreases. During the course of the day, the height of the disks varies by about 1% of the entire body height. Thus, a body height of 180 cm would show a variation of about 18 mm. In everyday activities, weight load and muscle tension lead to a reduction in the height of the disk. In a reclined position, on the other hand, the osmotic pressure of the disks allows them to absorb fluid, and their height increases again, thus also increasing neural tension. For this reason, it is normal that the leg, back, and cranial nerve mobility test is harder to pass directly on rising than at the end of a working day. In order to start the day with full neurodynamic mobility, this should be exercised until the test can be passed in the morning.

7.12 Posterior Thigh Flexibility

▶ **Starting position.** Lie on your back so that your left buttock (**Fig. 7.67**, ①) and your left heel touch the frame of an open door. Place a pillow under your head if you cannot pass the chin tuck mobility and thoracic spine extension tests (pp. 70 and 73).

Test

Can you push your heel so far up the door frame (without tension or pain) and straighten your left leg so far that your left calf touches the door frame (**Fig. 7.67**, ②), while your right leg lies so flat that your right calf touches the floor (**Fig. 7.67**, ③)?

Exercise

Straighten your left knee until you feel the onset of tension. Remain in this position until the tension resolves.

▶ **Alternative exercise.** If tension does not resolve during the exercise because the roots of the sciatic nerve are pinched in the lumbar spine, bending the lumbar spine to the opposite side may help to eliminate the tension (**Fig. 7.68**).

> **Lumbar dissociation**
>
> During the exercise you may keep your lumbar spine actively arched until it just begins to rise from the mat, in order to:
> - Increase the tension at the backs of the thighs
> - Unload the posterior aspect of the lumbar disks and provide muscular stabilization for hypermobile portions of the lumbar spine and the sacroiliac joints

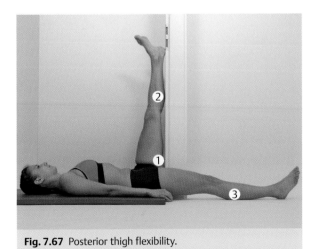

Fig. 7.67 Posterior thigh flexibility.

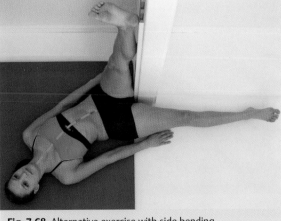

Fig. 7.68 Alternative exercise with side bending.

Troubleshooting

If the tension does not diminish over the course of the exercise, the following tests and exercises should be used to detect and resolve possible mechanical impediments. If one of the following tests is positive, have your patient do the corresponding exercise and then repeat the posterior thigh flexibility exercise. If the tension has now resolved, you have found and solved the blockade.

- Repeat the exercise with less tension while simultaneously doing all the relaxation exercises (pp. 39–49)
- Buttock muscle flexibility (p. 96)
- Leg, back, and cranial nerve mobility (p. 98)
- Hip extension mobility (p. 109)
- Anterior thigh flexibility (p. 113)
- Calf flexibility (p. 103)
- Back muscle strength (p. 118)
- Alternative exercise with lateral flexion (**Fig. 7.68**)

Before and After Comparison

How great is the distance between the left calf and the door frame, and how great is the distance between the right calf and the floor (**Fig. 7.69**)?

The distance is measured from the point on the calf that would touch the wall or the floor first if the patient had full mobility. This point can easily be determined if, before the test, the patient lies in the supine test position and stretches out both legs together on the floor. The point of the calf that touches the floor first (**Fig. 7.70**) is the point from which the distance to the door frame and the floor is measured in the test.

Add together the distance from the left calf to the door frame and the distance of the right calf from the floor. In addition to this number, document which leg was up against the door frame. In the test pictured (see **Fig. 7.67**), the record would be "L0" since the left leg (L) is on the door frame and the calves are completely touching the door

frame and the floor, respectively. If the right leg were against the door frame and the calves were each two fingers widths (F) from the goal, the record would be "R4F."

Differential Diagnosis

Whether symptoms arising during this exercise are caused by neurodynamic or myofascial tension may be determined as described under "Differential Diagnosis" for the leg, back, and cranial nerve mobility exercise (p. 100).

An indication of neural tension is a feeling of tension in the lumbar spine or the left shin during the exercise for left posterior thigh flexibility. A lessening of these symptoms when using the alternative exercise with right lateral flexion of the lumbar spine (see **Fig. 7.68**) indicates a neurodynamic blockade in the left lumbar foramina.

During the stretch of the left hamstring, a pulling sensation might be felt in the right groin and/or the right calf might not touch the floor (**Fig. 7.69**). Whether these findings are caused by a tightness of the right iliopsoas muscle can be verified by doing the hip extension mobility test (p. 109).

Biomechanics

Free ischiocrural mobility prevents hypermobility of the subsequent joints in the kinetic flexion chain, namely the sacroiliac joint and the L5–S1 segment. Whenever the hip is flexed, free ischiocrural mobility also decreases the load on the L5–S1 disk, which, at 58%, is by far the most frequently affected by herniation of the lumbar disks, compared with 36% for the L4–L5 disk and 5% for the L3–L4 disk (Schäfer 2005).

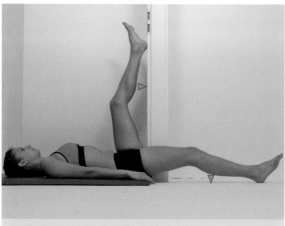

Fig. 7.69 The distance of the calves from the door frame and the floor.

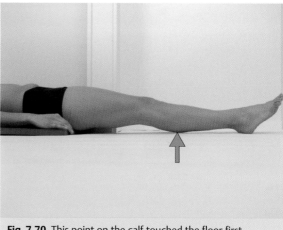

Fig. 7.70 This point on the calf touched the floor first.

7.13 Calf Flexibility

▶ **Starting position.**   Stand barefoot, facing a wall, on a hard floor (without a gym mat). Position your feet two foot lengths away from the wall, and point your toes straight forward. Take a step forward with your right foot so that the toes of your right foot and your right knee touch the wall (**Fig. 7.71**, ①). If you have done everything correctly, the distance between your right heel and your left toes is now one foot length (**Fig. 7.71**, ②). Turn your left foot inward until the outer edge of your left foot is perpendicular to the wall (**Fig. 7.72**). Now place your crossed forearms against the wall and lean your forehead against your forearms. Keep your pelvis parallel to the wall. Finally, without letting your left sole slip on the floor, turn your left knee outward as far as possible. If you do this correctly, the inner edge of your left foot will rise and your weight will be transferred to the outer edge of the foot, while the toes of the left foot will still be pointing straight forward.

Test

Can you straighten your left knee completely (without tension or pain) (see **Fig. 7.71**,) while your weight remains on the outer edge of your left foot?

> **Stabilizing the arch of the foot**
>
> Effective stretching of the calf and strengthening of the arch both require the arch of the foot to be maintained during the exercise.

Exercise

Straighten your left knee until you feel the onset of tension. Remain in this position until the tension resolves.

▶ **Alternative exercise.**   In addition to turning the left knee outward and shifting your body weight to the outer edge of the left foot, flexing your left toes as if they were grabbing a towel adds muscular stability to the arch of your foot.

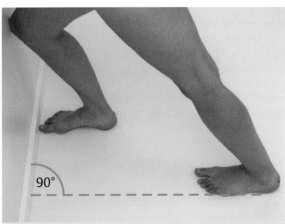

Fig. 7.72 The outer edge of your left foot should be perpendicular to the wall.

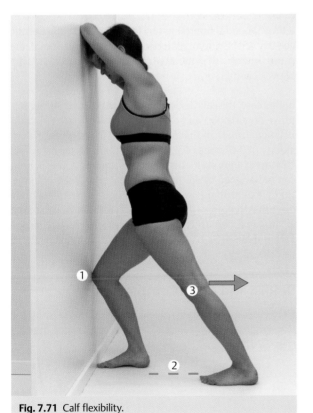

Fig. 7.71 Calf flexibility.

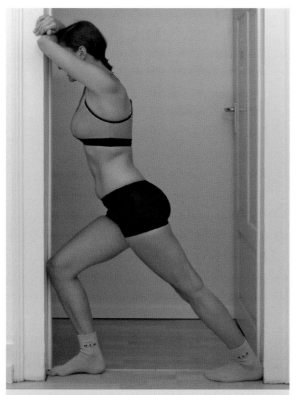

Fig. 7.73 Stretching the calves in the door frame avoids the danger of slipping on a smooth floor.

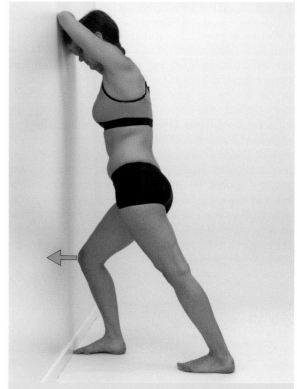

Fig. 7.74 The distance between the knee and the wall.

If you are standing on a smooth floor and do not want to take off your socks, you can also do the exercise in a door frame (**Fig. 7.73**) to avoid slipping. In this case, the front knee touches the door frame on one side while the heel of the back foot touches the door frame on the opposite side. In this way, you will not slip in spite of a smooth floor. If the width of the door happens to be three foot lengths, it can also be used for testing.

Troubleshooting

If the tension does not diminish over the course of the exercise, the following tests and exercises should be used to detect and resolve possible mechanical impediments. If one of the following tests is positive, have your patient do the corresponding exercise and then repeat the calf stretch. If the tension has now resolved, you have found and solved the blockade.
- Repeat the exercise with less tension while simultaneously doing all the relaxation exercises (p. 39)
- Anterior thigh flexibility (p. 113)
- Buttock muscle flexibility (p. 96)
- Leg, back, and cranial nerve mobility (p. 98)
- Posterior thigh flexibility (p. 101)

If dorsiflexion is limited not by the elastic resistance of the calf but because of hypomobility of the talocrural joint, the cause is often a degenerative change in the joint as a result of overloading, sprain, or fracture.

In this case, the calf flexibility exercise will usually not improve dorsiflexion and can even trigger irritation. A manual mobilization of the talocrural joint in the unloaded position (p. 145, see **Fig. 11.6**) is then a more useful treatment option. If this improves mobility, the patient can be assigned to do the calf flexibility exercise at home, to the extent that it is possible without pain, to maintain the improved dorsal extension. Often the talocrural joint is already so seriously damaged after a fracture or severe sprain that only a partial improvement in movement can be achieved.

Before and After Comparison

How great is the distance between the right knee and the wall when the first feeling of tension or blockade appears (**Fig. 7.74**)?

Differential Diagnosis

▶ **Joint blockade.** If dorsal extension is not limited by elastic tension of the calf muscles but by a blockade of the talocrural joint, this is usually felt by a narrowly localized sensation of pinching in the anterior joint line. After successful manual mobilization of the blockade, the pinching feeling disappears, and with the increased dorsiflexion, elastic tension is again felt in the calf.

▶ **Soleus vs. gastrocnemius.** If the test position for calf flexibility on the left (**Fig. 7.71**) triggers symptoms in the left calf, it can be determined whether they are caused by tension in the soleus or the gastrocnemius muscle by flexing and extending the left knee:
- If the symptoms increase with *knee extension*, the cause is tension in the *gastrocnemius*.
- If the cause is tension in the *soleus*, the symptoms increase when the *knee is flexed* without raising the heel (**Fig. 7.75**).

Soleus

If the soleus is too short, a heel lift and/or subtalar joint pronation is the typical compensatory movement that may be observed during the lifting technique test (p. 93).

Another way to distinguish between tightness of the gastrocnemius versus the soleus in the test position for calf flexibility (**Fig. 7.71**) is as follows. If the patient reports tension in the left calf (the back leg with the knee extended), this is a sign of tightness of the gastrocnemius. If she feels tension in the calf of the front leg with the knee flexed, tightness in the soleus is the probable cause.

Gastrocnemius

Tightness of the gastrocnemius is far more common than tightness of the soleus.

▶ **Reflex hypertonia.** Pain in the calf can be caused by reflex hypertonia due to an electrolyte imbalance or irritation of the tibial nerve (L4–S3). *Electrolyte imbalances* are most frequently associated with metabolic disorders or persistent heavy perspiration. In the practice of physical therapy, nerve irritation is a far more common finding.

▶ **Nerve irritation.** Nerve irritation can be caused by tension or compression. Increased tension or irritability of the tibial nerve is indicated when the calf symptoms in the test position for leg, back, and cranial nerve mobility (p. 98) decrease with extension of the cervical spine. In this case, leg, back, and cranial nerve mobility should be exercised and restored.

Narrow passages at which tibial nerve fibers from L4–S3 are often compressed are found at intervertebral foramina L4–L5 and L5–S1 in the spinal canal or under the pirifor-

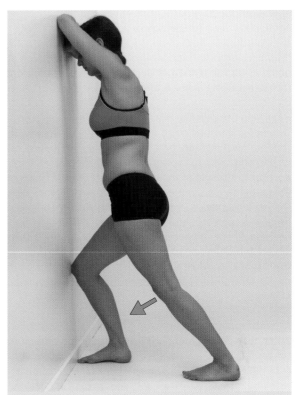

Fig. 7.75 Flexion of the left knee while the left heel remains on the floor.

mis muscle. Axial traction of the spine for 5 minutes will produce a significant reduction in the symptoms of *foraminal impingement*, but will fail to improve the symptoms of a spinal stenosis. Impingements due to lumbar spinal stenosis and some types of foraminal impingement are immediately reduced when the patient sits down. In a standing position, they can be improved gradually, from month to month, as the need for compensatory hyperlordosis of the lumbar spine decreases, due to an improvement in hip extension mobility (p. 109) and thoracic extension mobility (p. 73). Symptoms caused by nerve pinching under a hypertonic or shortened *piriformis* muscle decrease as soon as the muscle tension decreases during practice of the buttock muscle flexibility exercise (p. 96).

▶ **Overstressed calf and Achilles tendon.** Causes of an overstressed calf and Achilles tendon can be tight calf muscles, overtraining, a forefoot-striking style of running, or a gait pattern with externally rotated feet. The latter should only be corrected if the origin is not increased lateral torsion of the tibia or retroversion of the femoral neck.

Correction of a gait pattern with excessive external hip rotation requires free calf flexibility and buttock muscle flexibility (pp. 103 and 96). When these are present or have been regained, a physiological gait again becomes possible. While some patients then return to their physiological gait spontaneously, others need gait training in order to break their compensatory pattern.

If athletes overuse their Achilles tendon, a thickening or notch along the tendon or decreased lateral mobility of the retrocalcaneal bursa is often palpable.

▶ **Leg vein thrombosis.** Finally, where there is calf pain, a thrombosis must be ruled out. Indications of this condition are swelling and heat distal to the thrombosis, as well as sensitivity to pressure along the affected vein, frequently on the sole of the foot and between the heads of the gastrocnemius. If there are signs of acute thrombosis, the patient's physician should be immediately consulted on how to proceed. Mobilization of the calf should only be initiated after obtaining the physician's approval. Usually, mobilization can take place 2 weeks after the onset of the thrombosis, when the thrombus is tightly adherent to the vessel wall and can no longer dislodge to become an embolus.

▶ **Compartment syndrome.** Local trauma or chronic exertion may cause pronounced tenderness and tension in the respective compartment of the calf, or more frequently in the compartment of the anterior tibialis. If compartment syndrome is suspected, the patient's physician should be informed immediately.

Biomechanics

Free calf flexibility decreases the stress on the spine by permitting a physiological gait and lifting pattern. The calf flexibility exercise is intended to correct the typical imbalance of a shortened calf and fallen arch by simultaneously stretching the calf and raising the arch. Actively raising the arch strengthens the supporting muscles, prevents stretching of the supporting ligaments during the exercise, and reduces the elastic resistance in precisely those fibers of the calf muscle whose tightness resists the raising of the arch.

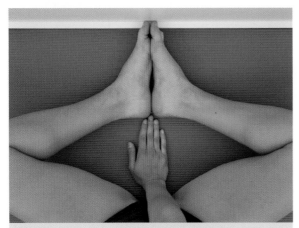

Fig. 7.76 The distance from the heel to the groin.

7.14 Inner Thigh Flexibility

▶ **Starting position.** Sit on the floor, facing a wall with the soles of your feet touching each other, the length of a hand between your groin and your heels (**Fig. 7.76**), and the tips of your feet touching the wall. Now lie on your back (**Fig. 7.77**). Place a pillow under your head if you are not able to pass the cervical and thoracic spine extension tests (pp. 70 and 73).

Test

> **Pain-free**
>
> As always, in the following steps 1 to 3, you should stay in the pain-free range and only go as far as the first feeling of tension.

Step 1: Can you part your knees until your lateral ankle bones touch the floor on either side (**Fig. 7.77**) without sliding away from the wall?

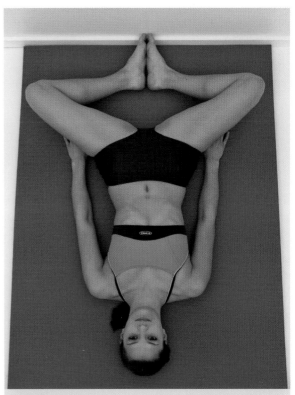

Fig. 7.77 Test step 1.

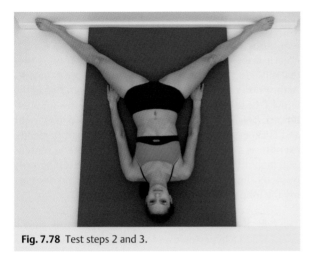

Fig. 7.78 Test steps 2 and 3.

Step 2: Can you now extend your legs on the floor with your heels against the wall (**Fig. 7.78**)?

Step 3: In this position (**Fig. 7.78**), can you push your lumbar spine down until it touches the floor?

Exercise

Do steps 1 to 3 until you feel the onset of tension. Remain in this position until the tension resolves.

▶ **Alternative exercise.** If the muscles of the interior thigh are so tight that you cannot fully extend your knees in the second part of the test (**Fig. 7.79**), slide away from the wall until you can fully extend your knees. With increasing mobility, you will need to slide away from the wall less and less.

Troubleshooting

If the tension does not diminish over the course of the exercise, the following tests and exercises should be used to detect and resolve possible mechanical impediments. If one of the following tests is positive, have your patient do the corresponding exercise and then repeat the inner thigh flexibility exercise. If the tension has now resolved, you have found and solved the blockade.

- Repeat the exercise with less tension while simultaneously doing all the relaxation exercises (p. 39)
- Hip extension mobility (p. 109)
- Thoracic extension mobility (p. 73)
- Anterior thigh flexibility (p. 113)
- Standing posture with a balanced upper body (p. 36)
- Seated posture with a balanced upper body (p. 25)

Before and After Comparison

Step 1: How great is the distance between each of the lateral ankle bones and the floor? The distances of the left and right lateral ankles from the floor should be added together.

Step 2: How many finger widths fit between the calf and the floor on the right and left sides (**Fig. 7.79**)?

The distance is measured from the point on the calf that would touch the floor first if the patient were able to fully extend her legs. This point can easily be determined if the patient lies on her back without contact with the wall and stretches out both legs close to each other on the floor. The point of the calf that touches the floor first (**Fig. 7.80**) is the point from which the distance to the floor is measured in the subsequent test.

Step 3: Does the lumbar spine touch the floor or not?

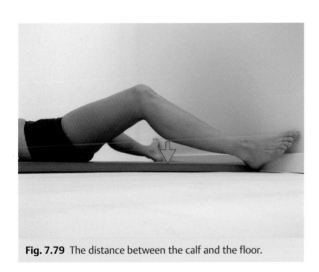

Fig. 7.79 The distance between the calf and the floor.

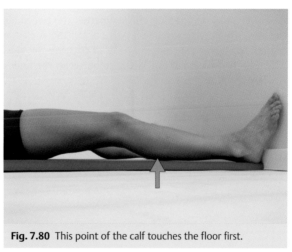

Fig. 7.80 This point of the calf touches the floor first.

Differential Diagnosis

▶ **Impingement.** A pinching sensation in step 1 of the exercise indicates degenerative changes or a dysfunction of the hip joint. The most frequently occurring dysfunction is anterior migration of the femoral head. If your patient experiences a pinching feeling in the groin in step 1 of the inner thigh flexibility exercise (see **Fig. 7.77**) and you wish to determine whether this is caused by anterior migration of the femoral head, stop the exercise and have your patient do the hip extension mobility exercise (p. 109). If you now repeat the inner thigh flexibility exercise, the pinching feeling in the groin caused by anterior migration of the femoral head should be immediately lessened or have completely gone.

If the pinching feeling experienced during the inner thigh flexibility exercise recurs after a short time, you have not yet eliminated the cause of the anterior femoral head migration. A further possible cause is a posture associated with tensing of the anterior muscle chain, including the iliopsoas muscle, such as an anterior pelvic shift (p. 36), or a seated posture with upper body leaning backward (p. 25). The cause of these postures, on the other hand, is often decreased thoracic extension mobility (p. 73).

Other causes of impingement are habitual sitting for extended periods (p. 51), a seat that is too low (p. 28), a seated posture in which the heels are not touching the floor (p. 30), or frequent work with a foot pedal, such as in the work of professional drivers or dentists.

If one of these postures or activities is responsible for a recurrent pinching feeling in the groin, daily and consistent correction should bring about gradual and permanent improvement.

▶ **Tension.** Tension in the interior thigh in step 2 indicates insufficient flexibility in the hip adductors.

If the elastic resistance of the hip adductors in step 2 is clearly stronger on one side, check whether the two sides are used asymmetrically in everyday activities. A classic example of this is the common habit of crossing the legs, which is checked for in the "distance between the knees and between the feet test" (p. 29).

Pubic symphysis

Especially with hip adductor hypertonicity after a fall, a blow to the pelvis, or vaginal birth, it should be checked whether there is a dysfunction of the pubic symphysis.

Biomechanics

▶ **Anterior migration of the femoral head.** A typical muscular imbalance in the hip area consists of weak gluteal muscles and a hypertonic and short iliopsoas muscle. Among other things, this leads to anterior migration of the femoral head from its central position when the hip is extended. This eccentric position leads to early joint wear and is experienced in step 1 of the inner thigh flexibility exercise as a pinching feeling in the groin. The hip extension mobility exercise corrects this imbalance temporarily by increasing the tone of the gluteal muscles and decreasing the tone of the iliopsoas muscle.

Two typical causes of the imbalance between weak gluteal muscles and a hypertonic and short iliopsoas muscle are a standing posture with an anterior pelvic shift and a seated posture with a backward-leaning upper body. Because the vector of gravity of the upper body runs behind the pivot at the hip joint in these two postures, it creates a hip extension torque that must be compensated for by sustained contraction of the hip flexors, including the iliopsoas muscle.

Another cause of muscular imbalance is regular sitting for long periods, because in this position the gluteal muscles are hypotonic and elongated, whereas the iliopsoas muscle is slack and thus prone to shortening.

▶ **Adductor stretching by hip extension.** Since most adductors originate relatively far anteriorly on the pubic bone, whereas their attachment is to the dorsal surface of the femur, they also act as hip flexors from the neutral position of the hip joint. For this reason, they can be additionally stretched, if, along with the hip adduction in step 2, hip extension is added via the pelvic tilt in step 3.

7.15 Hip Extension Mobility

▶ **Starting position.** Stand with your back against the inner side of a door frame. Take a step backward with your left foot passed the door frame so that your left heel and your left inner ankle are situated at the side of the door frame (**Fig. 7.81**, ①). Place your right foot flat on a chair in front of you. Your right leg should remain relaxed. Without raising either heel, tilt your pelvis so that your lumbar spine is firmly pressed against the door frame (**Fig. 7.81**, ②).

Test

Can you extend your left knee completely backward (without tension or pain) (**Fig. 7.81**, ③) while your lumbar spine maintains its initial firm pressure against the door frame (**Fig. 7.81**, ②)?

Exercise

Keep your lumbar spine firmly pressed against the door frame (**Fig. 7.81**, ②) while you extend your left knee (**Fig. 7.81**, ③) until you notice a resistance or a first stretch in your left groin. Remain in this position until the stretch and/or resistance in your left groin has decreased. The quadriceps muscle at the front of your left thigh, on the other hand, must remain contracted in order to maintain this stretching position.

▶ **Alternative exercise.** As soon as you master the sequence of movements in the exercise, you will be able to do the exercise without a wall: you can just imagine one. Once you no longer need a wall, you can place your right foot on any convenient elevation, for example the second step of a staircase.

Troubleshooting

If the tension does not diminish over the course of the exercise, the following tests and exercises should be used to detect and resolve possible mechanical impediments. If one of the following tests is positive, have your patient do the corresponding exercise and then repeat the hip extension mobility exercise. If the tension has now resolved, you have found and solved the blockade.
- Repeat the exercise with less tension while simultaneously doing all the relaxation exercises (p. 39)
- Anterior thigh flexibility (p. 113)
- Manual release technique for the psoas muscle and the iliacus muscle (p. 145, see **Figs. 11.4** and **11.5**)

Groin pain caused by an inguinal hernia usually does not change as a result of the hip extension mobility exercise. If groin pain is increased by the exercise, the tension should be reduced enough so that this does not happen again. Usually, the exercise does bring relief of hip symptoms, even in the case of inguinal hernia, probably be-

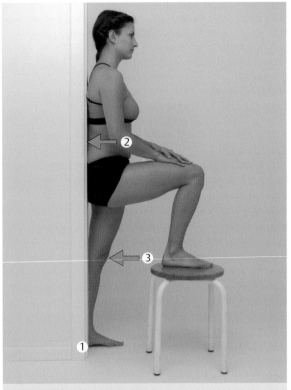

Fig. 7.81 Hip extension mobility.

cause some part of the symptoms is due to some other causes (see "Differential Diagnosis" for this section) that can be corrected by the exercise. After surgical repair of an inguinal hernia, consult with the surgeon as to whether and to what extent hip extension mobility may be exercised.

In cases of severe degenerative changes of the hip, a disposition toward inflammatory reactions, and age above 80, hip extensor mobility often cannot be improved. But because there are always exceptions, even in these cases, it is worthwhile making a gentle attempt after explaining to the patient that the exercise may produce a temporary increase in her hip symptoms.

Before and After Comparison

Have your patient take the starting position of the hip extension mobility exercise without pressing her lumbar spine against the wall. Instead, ask her to lean on her right thigh with her forearms, and extend her left knee backward as far as she can (**Fig. 7.82**). Now place your extended right hand with your fingertips against the door frame, with the radial side of your index finger touching the back of the patient's knee (**Fig. 7.83**). Then ask the patient to press her lumbar spine firmly against the door frame and extend her left knee as far as possible without a feeling of tension in the groin and without decreasing the pressure of the lumbar spine against the door frame (**Fig. 7.84**). How great a distance does this leave between the radial side of the index finger and the back of the patient's left knee (**Fig. 7.85**)?

Differential Diagnosis

▶ Iliopsoas

Iliopsoas

Tightness and hypertonicity of the iliopsoas muscle are the most frequent causes of restricted hip joint extension mobility.

Typical reasons for tightness and hypertonicity of the iliopsoas are a sedentary lifestyle, too little exercise, too much sitting (p. 51), a standing posture with an anterior pelvic shift (p. 36), a seated posture with crossed or adducted legs (p. 29), sitting on a seat that is too low (p. 28), sitting with the heels raised (p. 30), sitting with the upper body inclined backward (p. 25), or frequent work with a foot pedal, such as in the work of professional drivers or dentists.

Overexerting the iliopsoas in this manner may cause it to become painful. In addition, tightness of the iliopsoas muscle can lead to anterior migration of the femoral head. The resulting dysfunction of the hip joint often causes the type of groin pain that may be triggered by step 1 of the inner thigh flexibility test (see **Fig. 7.77**).

▶ **Hernias.** Groin pain caused by an inguinal or femoral hernia, on the other hand, cannot be modified by this test. However, because of reflex guarding, this pain may cause tightness and hypertonicity of the iliopsoas.

The inguinal hernia is the most frequently occurring hernia; 90% of these occur in men. Where abdominal content such as the peritoneum or portions of the intestine descend through the inguinal canal, the hernia projects through the abdominal wall immediately *above* the inguinal ligament, and may extend as far as into the testicles. In addition to groin symptoms, this can lead to pain and visible enlargement of the ipsilateral testicle. Rarely do hernias appear in women, and if so, they are usually femoral hernias. In this case, they pass through the abdominal wall directly *below* the inguinal ligament and medial to the femoral vein.

If the hernia bulges visibly when the abdominal pressure increases in response to sneezing, the Valsalva maneuver, or raising the head in the supine position, the diagnosis is easy. Often, however, hernias are neither visible nor palpable, which complicates the diagnosis. In such cases, signs such as an increase in the symptoms with sneezing are an indication, although they are not always reproducible due to the variable location of the abdominal tissue.

In the case of a so-called "strangulated hernia," the abdominal contents are pinched in the hernia, which leads to ischemia and tissue necrosis. When this occurs, the pain increases rapidly, sometimes accompanied by fever, and the situation is life-threatening. Therefore, signs of a strangulated hernia require immediate medical attention.

Biomechanics

Restricted hip extensor mobility can result in compensatory hyperextension and overloading of the lumbar spine (Link et al 1990, Piper 2005).

For this reason, the improvement of a hip extension deficit is especially important in patients whose lower back pain increases when the hips are extended, that is, when standing, in the supine position with the legs extended, or in the prone position, whereas they decrease in the sitting or supine position with the hips bent. In this case, patients' lower back pain is best prevented by doing the hip extension mobility exercise immediately before activities requiring a repeated or continuous hip extension.

In addition to improving hip extension mobility, this exercise also strengthens the abdominal muscles and the hip extensors as they tilt the pelvis. This corrects the typical imbalance of a shortened and hypertonic iliopsoas muscle on one side, and weak, overstretched hip extensors and abdominal muscles on the other side.

Weak antagonists

Where the imbalance is pronounced, it may take several training sessions until the abdominal muscles and hip extensors have become sufficiently strong to generate a stretch of the strong iliopsoas muscle that the patient can feel.

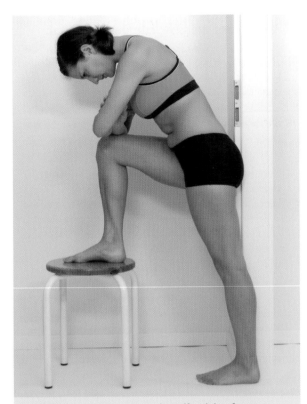

Fig. 7.82 The patient supports herself with her forearms on her right thigh, and extends her left knee completely.

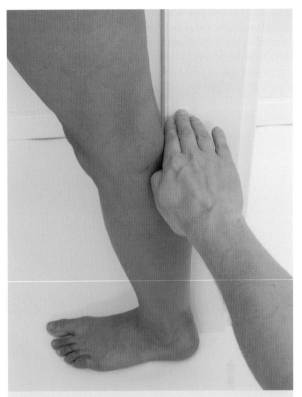

Fig. 7.83 The therapist marks this knee position with his hand.

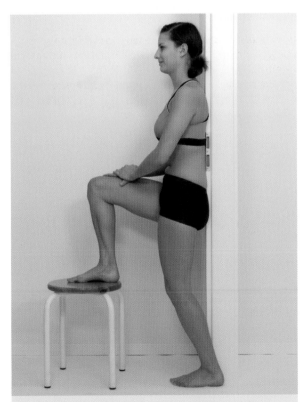

Fig. 7.84 In the following test of hip extension mobility …

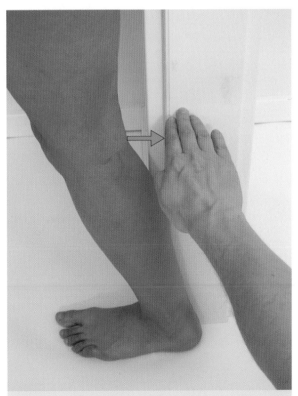

Fig. 7.85 … the distance between the therapist's index finger and the back of the patient's knee is measured.

If no effect of exercise is felt at first, the patient may doubt the efficacy of the exercise and may therefore lack the motivation to do it. To prevent this, you can enable your patient to feel a noticeable effect by having her do the following awareness exercise immediately before and after the hip extension mobility exercise.

Awareness exercise: Lumbar relaxation

Lie on your back with your legs outstretched. Now pay attention to how your lumbar spine feels. Feel with your lumbar spine, not with your hands. Does your lumbar spine feel comfortable and relaxed, or do you feel any unpleasant tension? Try to imagine how far your lumbar arch rises from the floor. Finally, feel how great the distance and the elastic resistance are that you must overcome in order to press your lumbar spine to the floor.

Now do the hip extension mobility exercise once. Make sure you do it thoroughly. Then lie on the floor again. See whether your lumbar spine now feels different, and whether the distance and the elastic resistance that you must overcome so that you can press your lumbar spine to the floor have changed.

You will probably feel that your lumbar arch is significantly flatter and more relaxed following the hip extension mobility exercise. This relaxation improves the blood flow to your back muscles and unloads your disks. If you sleep with your legs extended and improve your hip extensor mobility immediately before going to bed, you will profit from this effect all night long.

7.16 Anterior Thigh Flexibility

▶ **Starting position.** Kneel without shoes on the floor with your knees the width of two fists apart. Your extended toes should be lying on the floor with the toenails facing down. Your great toes should be crossed. The distance between your great toes and the wall should equal two fist widths (**Fig. 7.86**, ①). Sit on your heels and lean your shoulders and head against the wall. Behind your back, grasp the opposite forearm with each hand as close to the elbow as possible, and keep both forearms in contact with your back (**Fig. 7.87**, ②). Make sure that your knees stay firmly pressed to the floor. Finally, tilt your pelvis so that your lumbar spine is pressed toward the wall (**Fig. 7.88**, ③), while you continue to sit on your heels.

Test

Can you press your lumbar spine toward the wall (without tension or pain) (**Fig. 7.88**, ③), until one of your fingers (**Fig. 7.87**, ④) touches the wall?

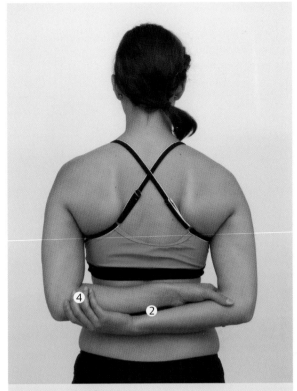

Fig. 7.87 Locked forearms.

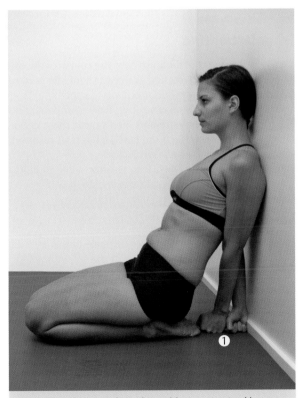

Fig. 7.86 A distance of two fist widths is maintained between toes and the wall.

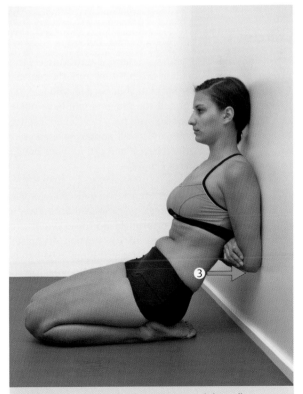

Fig. 7.88 Pressing the lumbar spine toward the wall.

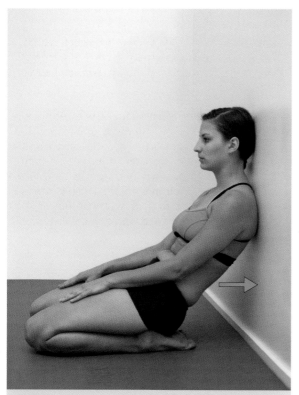

Fig. 7.89 Exercise for anterior thigh flexibility without locked arms.

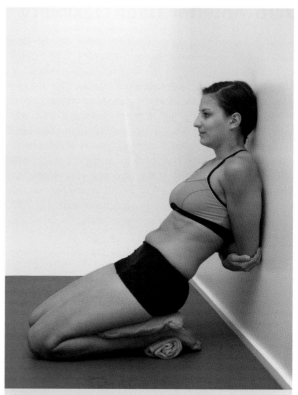

Fig. 7.90 A cushion and a rolled-up towel help with unpleasant tension in the knees and back of the feet.

Exercise

Press your lumbar spine toward the wall until you feel the onset of tension. Remain in this position until the tension resolves. The locked forearms at your back let you feel the direction of movement and the progress you have made with the exercise. As soon as you have developed a sense for both these parameters, you will no longer need your arms behind you for the exercise and can let your hands lie loosely on your thighs (**Fig. 7.89**).

▶ **Alternative exercise.** If the tension in your knees or the back of your feet is too great, place a cushion between your heels and buttocks, or a rolled-up towel under the backs of your feet (**Fig. 7.90**). As the tension decreases with time, you can use increasingly thinner towel rolls and cushions until at some point you may no longer need them.

Troubleshooting

If the tension does not diminish over the course of the exercise, the following tests and exercises should be used to detect and resolve possible mechanical impediments. If one of the following tests is positive, have your patient do the corresponding exercise and then repeat the anterior thigh flexibility exercise. If the tension has now resolved, you have found and solved the blockade.
- Repeat the exercise with less tension while simultaneously doing all the relaxation exercises (p. 39)
- Hip extension mobility (p. 109)
- Posterior thigh flexibility (p. 101)

The most frequently encountered obstacle in the anterior thigh flexibility exercise is cramps in the sole of the foot. They are caused by plantar flexion hypomobility and can easily be avoided with an adequately thick roll under the instep (**Fig. 7.90**). With regular exercise, the height of the roll can be reduced every week until a roll is no longer needed. Once complete plantar flexion mobility is regained in this way, it can be maintained with a little exercise.

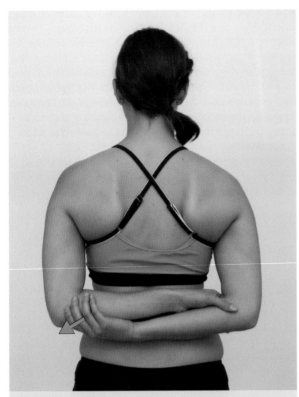

Fig. 7.91 The distance of the fingers from the wall (blue arrow) is measured.

Before and After Comparison

How great is the distance between the wall and the fingers that are grasping the forearm (**Fig. 7.91**)?

Differential Diagnosis

▶ **Meniscal damage.** If the anterior thigh flexibility exercise is done without a cushion between the buttocks and the heels, the knee is flexed to the end of its range, which stresses the posterior horn of the meniscus. An intact meniscus can tolerate this without difficulty. If, however, a patient with a tear in the posterior horn of the meniscus gets into the starting position of the anterior thigh flexibility exercise, she will typically feel an intense pain in the knee and thigh that is hard to localize and is increased rather than decreased by holding the position.

The painful range of knee flexion should then be blocked with a cushion between the heels and the buttocks (see **Fig. 7.90**) so that the knee extensors stop their muscle guarding and may relax over the course of the exercise.

Posterior horn of the meniscus

The anterior thigh flexibility exercise cannot repair the meniscus problem, but by relaxing the rectus femoris muscle, it serves to prevent dysfunction further up the kinetic chain.

▶ **Patella.** A patellofemoral dysfunction with retropatellar cartilage degeneration can also cause an intense pain in the knee and thigh that is hard to localize and increases rather than decreases when the stretching position is held. In contrast to meniscal damage, the pain in the stretching position is felt more in the anterior region of the knee and decreases to the extent that the patellofemoral dysfunction is improved with physical therapy.

Patellofemoral joint

Carrying out the anterior thigh flexibility exercise over a pain-free range can produce a noticeable improvement of patellofemoral function in everyday activities.

▶ **Sacroiliac joint.** If limited flexibility of the rectus femoris muscle is the cause of the dysfunction in the sacroiliac joint, the feeling of tension encountered in the anterior thigh flexibility exercise is usually more intense on one side than the other and releases quite quickly. With the release, there is an immediate improvement in the sacroiliac dysfunction and pain that was caused by the muscle tension. This response distinguihses it from the muscle guarding of an impinged meniscus, where neither the dysfunction nor the associated muscle guarding improve with the anterior thigh flexibility exercise.

Biomechanics

▶ **Shoes.** The exercise should be done without shoes because shoes limit talocrural and subtalar mobility and may cause an unphysiological, compensatory twisting of the knee.

▶ **Cartilage.** As described under "Differential Diagnosis" in this section, muscle guarding of the quadriceps can be the result of a pain-induced flexion deficit in the knee. A typical underlying cause of this flexion deficit is a habit of sitting in chairs rather than squatting or sitting on the heels. As a result, the daily physiological loading in end range knee flexion, which keeps the surrounding tissue flexible and the cartilage resilient, is lacking.

As long as not all the cartilage is lost, it makes sense to foster cartilage regeneration by gradually increasing the knee flexion range by means of the anterior thigh flexibility exercise within a pain-free range.

Caution: After cruciate ligament reconstruction

No cruciate ligament reconstruction can match the original interlaced fiber structure. Depending on the surgical technique, postoperative end range knee flexion can therefore be temporarily or permanently contraindicated. This must be clarified with the surgeon before undertaking the anterior thigh flexibility exercise.

▶ **Patella.** An increase in patellofemoral contact pressure during the exercise is unavoidable. However, if the muscle relaxes as a result of the exercise, the contact pressure in subsequent everyday activities is less for an extended time, which contributes to recovery of the patellofemoral joint.

Vastus medialis

The anterior thigh flexibility exercise should never cause swelling in the knee because swelling causes a reflex inhibition, which affects the vastus medialis to a greater extent than the vastus lateralis, and thus, among other things, promotes patellofemoral dysfunction.

▶ **Sacroiliac joint.** In positions with hip extension and knee flexion (e.g., **Fig. 6.5** d), a tight rectus femoris muscle may pull the ipsilateral ilium into anterior rotation by means of its attachment to the anterior superior iliac spine. A bilateral tightness of the rectus femoris will tend to pull the entire pelvis, and thus also the lumbar spine into hyperlordosis. A unilateral tightness of the rectus femoris, on the other hand, promotes twisting of the sacroiliac joint. If the restricted flexibility of the rectus femoris is not promptly recognized and corrected by means of the anterior thigh flexibility test and exercise, the constant twisting of the ilium can lead to chronic irritation and instability in the sacroiliac joint.

8 Strength

This chapter contains only a few selected strength exercises because good posture, active mobility exercises, gravity, and our daily activities provide sufficient exercise for most muscles to keep us healthy. Except for competitive sports, additional strengthening of these muscles is thus rarely necessary, wastes time, and overloads the joints. If you have followed the proposed sequence of posture, relaxation, movement, coordination, and mobility in this book, you have already covered the most important aspects in respect to spinal health, and can now give your patient the final polish with the remaining strengthening and endurance exercises.

> ### Caution: Blood pressure
>
> In all the following strength exercises, avoid holding one's breath to prevent raising blood pressure excessively.

If your patient builds and maintains enough strength to pass the following strength tests even at the end of the working day, her muscles will be fit to support and move her spine safely throughout her day.

8.1 Abdominal and Anterior Neck Muscle Strength

▶ **Starting position.** Lie on your back with bent knees and your feet flat on the floor.

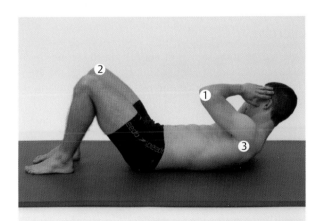

Fig. 8.1 Strengthening the abdominal and anterior neck muscles.

Press your lumbar spine flat to the floor with your fingertips at your temples. Push your neck backward, as described in the alternative exercise for chin tuck mobility (p. 71, **Fig. 7.5**) so that the distance between your neck and the floor gets smaller. Feel how this tightens the muscles at the front of your neck and moves your chin closer to your chest. Maintain this anterior neck muscle tension and the small chin to chest distance while performing slow, even movements to bring your head and your left elbow (**Fig. 8.1**, ①) toward your right knee (**Fig. 8.1**, ②) until your left shoulder blade (**Fig. 8.1**, ③) starts rising from the floor. Allow 3 seconds for this movement and then return to the starting position in another 3 seconds, just as slowly and evenly. Repeat this sequence, alternating between left and right.

Test

Can you perform this movement slowly, smoothly, and without trembling, pain, or considerable exertion, 10 times on each side?

Exercise

Repeat this movement along as you can do it slowly, smoothly, and without trembling, pain, or considerable exertion. A slow, regular movement is more effective and safe than a jolting jerk upward. Initially, it is useful to time yourself by whispering "one one thousand, two one thousand …" and to return to the starting position just as slowly, while inhaling. This helps you to become accustomed to the slow tempo and avoid an excessive rise in blood pressure. If this respiratory rhythm makes you dizzy or short of breath, you should stop the exercise and ask your therapist for advice.

> ### Awareness exercise: Symmetry
>
> Can you feel whether the movement is the same on both sides? Which parts of the body am I moving? How do I roll my thoracic vertebrae off the floor? Which muscles am I using? If you notice a difference between the two sides, try to "copy" the side that moves more smoothly.

▶ **Alternative exercise.** If the exercise with fingertips at the temples (**Fig. 8.1**) produces discomfort in the cervical spine, you should try to see whether this can be avoided by clasping your fingers behind your head in order to support its weight (**Fig. 8.2**).

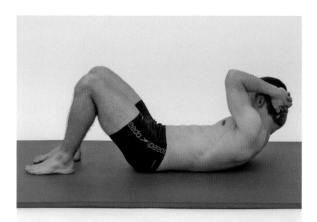

Fig. 8.2 The fingers are clasped behind the head.

Troubleshooting

If it is impossible to exercise in the supine position, the abdominal muscles can also be strengthened with alternative exercises (see **Figs. 10.9**, **10.10**, **10.11**). They can be more easily integrated into everyday activities, for instance at the office while telephoning; thus providing those patients with an exercise option, who would otherwise not find the time.

Before and After Comparison

How many repetitions can your patient do slowly, smoothly, and without trembling, pain, or considerable exertion?

Differential Diagnosis

If your patient's abdominal muscles are stronger on one side, she will tend to compensate on the weaker side by raising that shoulder by means of more thoracic rotation and less thoracic spine flexion. Therefore, a comparison of strength requires an observation of whether the mix of flexion and rotation of the thoracic spine is the same on both sides in the test and the exercise.

Biomechanics

Symmetrical abdominal and anterior neck muscle strength stabilizes the lumbar and cervical spine and prevents it from being hyperextended. In addition, it relaxes the antagonistic extensor muscles in these regions. This may explain why strong abdominal muscles reduce the incidence of back pain by about half (Hides et al 2001).

Tight abdominal muscles

There is a widespread belief that the spine benefits from keeping the abdominal muscles constantly tightened. This is not true. This kind of exaggerated continuous contraction prevents adequate perfusion and development of the muscles, overloads the vertebral segment, and, unbalances the equilibrium of the spinal muscles. A balanced and dynamic posture (pp. 25, 36, and 53) automatically provides an appropriate abdominal muscle tension that will increase and decrease rhythmically with abdominal breathing (p. 47); thus, stimulating the metabolism of the abdominal muscles like a pump.

8.2 Back Muscle Strength

▶ **Starting position.** Lie face down. Extend your arms and legs, and rest your forehead on the floor (**Fig. 8.3**). Until you pass the hip extension mobility test (p. 109), you should also place a cushion under your abdomen (**Fig. 8.4**) to avoid hyperextension of your lumbar spine.

Tip your pelvis so that your buttocks contract, your pubic bone is pressed to the floor, and overarching of your lumbar spine is prevented. Then raise your left arm and right leg only as far as is possible without decreasing the pressure of your pubic bone against the floor, and hold this position (see **Fig. 8.3**) for 10 seconds.

Alternate sides when repeating the exercise. So, for the second repetition, raise your right arm and left leg, and for the third repetition, your left arm and right leg, etc.

Test

Can you complete a total of 12 of these 10-second repetitions (6 per side), steadily, without pain, trembling, or considerable exertion?

Exercise

Hold the position shown in **Fig. 8.3** for 10 seconds each and keep alternating sides as long as you can do the exercise with control, steadily, and without pain, trembling, or considerable exertion.

Alternative Exercise

Place a cushion under your abdomen (**Fig. 8.4**), while doing the exercise, if you have not yet passed the hip extension mobility test (p. 109). This will enable you to stabilize your lumbar spine and keep it from arching too much, even if you have not yet regained full hip extension mobility.

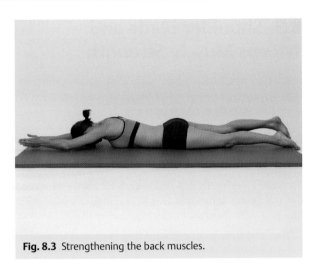

Fig. 8.3 Strengthening the back muscles.

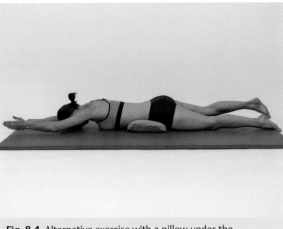

Fig. 8.4 Alternative exercise with a pillow under the abdomen.

Troubleshooting

If your patient is not sufficiently mobile to raise her arms and legs in this exercise without hyperextending her lumbar spine, she should place a cushion under her abdomen (**Fig. 8.4**). At the same time, the following tests and exercises should be used to detect and resolve possible mechanical impediments to hip, chest, and shoulder extension:

- Hip extension mobility (p. 109)
- Thoracic extension mobility (p. 73)
- Shoulder mobility (p. 78)
- Rotational mobility (p. 90)

If back muscle strengthening in the prone position proves to be impossible, the back muscles can also be strengthened with the shoulder blade and triceps muscle strength exercise (p. 120), with the thoracic extension mobility exercise (p. 73), and, last but not least, by maintaining a neutral spinal curvature (p. 12) in everyday activities.

Before and After Comparison

How many 10-second repetitions can your patient do steadily, without pain, trembling, or considerable exertion?

Differential Diagnosis

Scoliosis versus hypertrophy

If the erector spinae muscle seems more prominent on one side, it may, in fact, be hypertrophied. But it also may only seem so if the patient has scoliosis and the underlying vertebrae are twisted toward the convexity. This can be determined by visual inspection for rib prominence and the manual test of how far the relaxed erector spinae can be moved laterally when the patient is prone.

- Scoliosis: If prone, the lateral mobility of the erector spinae feels the same on both sides while in a stooped position an ipsilateral rib hump becomes visible in the same section of the spine, the muscle only appears hypertrophic because of the scoliotic rotation.
- Hypertrophy: If prone, the erector spinae feels hypertrophied and broader when the sides are compared, but no rib prominence becomes visible in stooped position, there actually is asymmetrical muscle growth.
- Scoliosis and hypertrophy: This asymmetrical muscle growth can have multiple causes, one being that on the convex side of a lateral spinal curvature, the muscles must work harder during sitting, standing, and walking to keep the superior sections of the body plumb. Thus, a muscle prominence in scoliosis can be caused by both rotation of the vertebrae and muscular hypertrophy.

Other causes of asymmetrical hypertrophy of the back extensors can be detected and corrected with the following tests and exercises:

- Symmetrical weight distribution when sitting (p. 30)
- Symmetrical weight distribution when standing (p. 33)
- Sitting without side bending or twisting (p. 21)
- Posture-friendly environment (p. 27)
- Arm nerve mobility (p. 83)
- Leg, back, and cranial nerve mobility (p. 98)

Biomechanics

Vertebral alignment

Symmetrical back muscle strength contributes significantly to repositioning rotated vertebrae and holding them in line.

This can be explained by the fact that muscles that attach symmetrically on both sides to a vertebra are slightly stretched on one side and slack on the other side due to rotation of the vertebra. Since a muscle can exert more force from a slightly stretched starting position than from a slack position, a bilateral contraction will turn the vertebra in the direction of the prestretched and thus more powerful muscle rather than its slack opposite, until the vertebra is repositioned and the muscles on both sides of the vertebra again have the same starting length.

The stabilizing function of the back extensors may be a reason why training of the multifidus muscles, together with co-contraction of the transverse abdominal muscles, clearly decreases the probability of new back pain episodes after 1 year (training group 30%, control group 84%) and 2 to 3 years (training group 35%, control group 75%), compared with the control group (Hides et al 2001).

An efficacious method for symmetrically strengthening the back extensors is an erect posture with neutral spinal curvature (p. 12). The loading of muscles in daily life is, however, rarely symmetrical, for instance due to handedness. Therefore it is useful to find and correct asymmetries in back muscle strength with the appropriate tests and exercises.

8.3 Shoulder Blade and Triceps Muscle Strength

▶ **Starting position.** Stand with your back against the wall with your heels one foot length away from the wall, your feet one shoe width apart (p. 32), and your knees slightly bent. Tilt your pelvis so that your lumbar lordosis flattens (as in the exercises to strengthen abdominal and back muscles, pp. 117 and 118), and hold this tilt while you push your pelvis forward slightly away from the wall. Turn the inner surface of your hands forward and spread out your arms somewhat (**Fig. 8.5 a**). Stick out your chest and pull your shoulder blades together until you feel how your muscles tighten between your shoulder blades. Then push your forearms into the wall until your upper arms and shoulders move forward only just far enough to lose contact with the wall and hold this position. *Only your forearms* should be in contact with the wall (**Fig. 8.5 b**) in this position, while your head, shoulders, upper arms, back, and buttocks no longer touch the wall.

Test

Can you hold this position steadily, without trembling, pain, or considerable exertion, for 60 seconds?

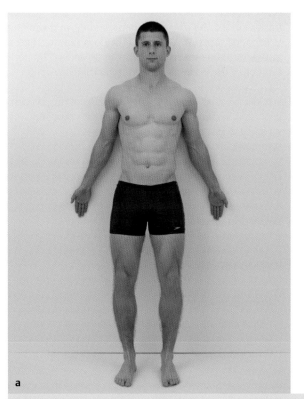
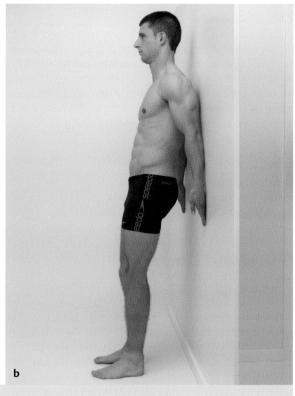

Fig. 8.5 Strengthening the shoulder blade and triceps muscles.

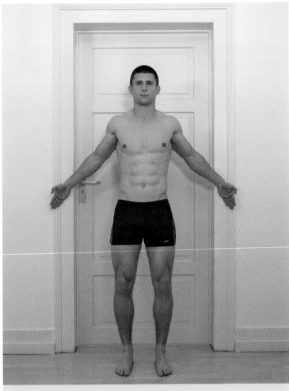

Fig. 8.6 Alternative exercise in the door frame.

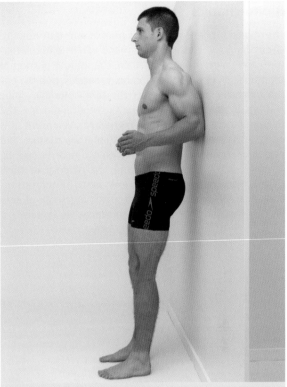

Fig. 8.7 Alternative exercise with the elbows bent.

Exercise

Hold the position shown in **Fig. 8.5**, as long as you can do so steadily, without trembling, pain, or considerable exertion.

▶ **Alternative exercises.** If you cannot find a free wall space for doing the exercise, you can brace your forearms against a door frame (**Fig. 8.6**).

Another, somewhat less strenuous variation, is to do the exercise with bent elbows. In this case, only the elbows, and not the forearms, touch the wall (**Fig. 8.7**).

Troubleshooting

If the exercise is too hard for beginners, it is possible to start with the feet closer to the wall.

Before and After Comparison

How many seconds can your patient maintain the position steadily, without trembling, pain, or considerable exertion?

Differential Diagnosis

Local hypertonicity of the finger flexors and extensors is a significant cause of tenosynovitis and epicondylitis. It is best resolved through smoothly coordinated activation of the entire hand–arm–shoulder–trunk muscle chain with emphasis on the proximal elements. The shoulder blade and triceps muscle strength exercise is suitable for this purpose, as is basketball or swimming.

Tenosynovitis and epicondylitis

If the symptoms have been caused by local hypertonicity of the finger flexors or extensors, they will not stop immediately with exercise. It can, however, be expected that symptoms will begin to decrease noticeably after 2 weeks of regular exercising.

If the lateral and medial heads of the triceps brachii are to be excluded from the test or training of shoulder blade and triceps muscle strength, the exercise can be repeated with the elbows bent to about 90° so that the elbows instead of the forearms are touching the wall (**Fig. 8.7**). However, it must be kept in mind that this shortens the lever arm for the shoulder muscles, automatically making the exercise easier.

Biomechanics

The shoulder blade and triceps muscle strength exercise strengthens the entire glenohumeral extension musculature, and down the muscle chain, the middle portion of the trapezius muscle, the rhomboid muscles, and the entire extension musculature of the thoracolumbar spine and hip. In the cervical spine, on the other hand, it is the flexion musculature that is strengthened. As a result, this one exercise manages to reverse numerous posture and muscle imbalances caused by habitually incorrect sitting postures. Most patients will find the reversal of their dysfunctional patterns with the exercise to be quite strenuous, but will be rewarded with a pleasant sense of ease and invigoration directly after performing the exercise.

Practicality

This strengthening exercise can easily be done in any office!

Since some of the muscles mentioned insert onto or arise at the spinous processes, the symmetrical strengthening exercises for shoulder blade and triceps muscle strength (p. 120) and back muscle strengthen (p. 118), help to reposition rotated vertebrae and stabilize their neutral position.

9 Endurance

Test

Do you train your endurance at least 3 × 30 minutes a week with your pulse constantly at about 120 beats per minute and still feel well at the end of the training?

Exercise

Train your endurance at least 3 × 30 minutes per week.

Work out at an intensity level at which your cardiovascular system remains active for 30 minutes, while on the other hand you still feel fine at the end of the training period. If you train your endurance with a goal of wellness and health, a constant pulse rate of 120 beats per minute is sufficient.

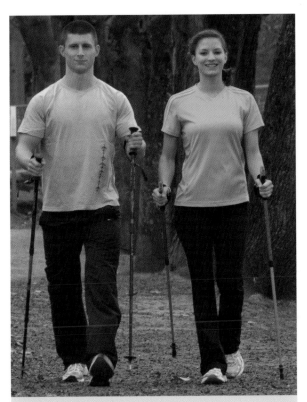

Fig. 9.1 Nordic walking as endurance training.

Heart rate monitor

If the traditional pulse measurement with a watch and palpation of the pulse is not your preferred method, you can also train with a heart rate monitor. Measurement devices of this type should, however, not lead you to focus solely on *numbers* and thus keep you from developing a *feeling* of what is good for you.

If this improves your well-being, you can gradually progress your cardiovascular workout from 3 × 30 minutes to a maximum of 3 × 60 minutes a week. More is not advisable, since it will tend to wear your joints in the long run.

If 30 minutes nonstop is too much at first, you should pause as often as necessary. For instance, if you decide to train by jogging but tire after 5 minutes, slow down to a walk for a while and only start jogging when you feel energetic again.

▶ **Alternative exercises.** Suitable endurance sports involve smooth, cyclical movements without excessive resistance or weight bearing. Examples are brisk walking (speed walking) with or without poles (Nordic walking, **Fig. 9.1**), dancing, cross-country skiing, jogging (**Fig. 9.2**), inline skating, aerobics, and, not least, swimming the crawl or back crawl. Since variation is good for the body, mixing sports is optimal, for instance swimming twice and dancing once a week.

Troubleshooting

When swimming the crawl, it is important to consider that the cervical spine can only relax when the face is submerged in the water during exhalation. In addition, swimming the crawl with a physiological shoulder and spine motion also requires free thoracic extension mobility (p. 73), rotational mobility (p. 90), shoulder mobility (p. 78), and hip extension mobility (p. 109).

Bicycling may be the ideal type of endurance training for a patient with an irreversible hip extension hypomobility or lumbar spine stenosis; for others it is not optimal because your patient is again sitting and is unable to move her spine freely. If she would like to bicycle in spite of these limitations, she should set her handlebars as high as possible so that she does not have to hyperextend her neck to keep her eyes on the road ahead.

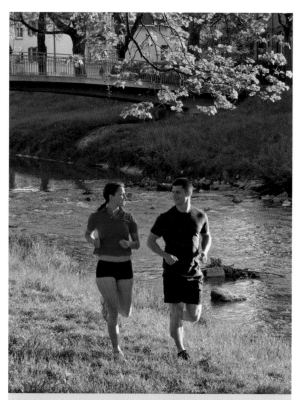

Fig. 9.2 Jogging as endurance training.

If a lack of time keeps your patient from regular endurance training, it might help to discuss with the patient what part of her daily route she can use as endurance training, for instance by occasionally riding a bicycle to work rather than driving every day. Even a brisk walk to work is endurance training that can easily be worked into the everyday routine of most patients. If the distance to work is too great for this, your patient, if she drives, can simply park her car a little farther away, or alternately get off a few stops further away if she uses public transportation.

Caution: Shortness of breath

If a patient sticks to the endurance training plan you have worked out for her and still experiences shortness of breath or discomfort at the slightest physical exertion, she should be examined by a cardiologist.

Before and After Comparison

How many minutes a week of endurance training does your patient perform with a pulse rate of 120 beats per minute and a subjective feeling of well-being?

Differential Diagnosis

The most frequent cause of chest pain in physical therapy practice is a blockade of the thoracic vertebrae or ribs. Heart problems such as angina pectoris are less often responsible.

▶ **Symptoms caused by blockade.** Symptoms of locked thoracic vertebrae or ribs can be triggered by thoracic spine or respiratory movements, but not by a rise of the pulse rate in response to cardiovascular exertion. In addition, symptoms caused by blockade clearly improve as soon as the blockade has been eliminated. This can be achieved by manual techniques, but often also with the following exercises:
- Rotational mobility (p. 90)
- Leg, back, and cranial nerve mobility (p. 98)
- Abdominal breathing (p. 47)
- Neutral spinal curvature (p. 12)
- Back muscle flexibility (p. 76)
- Thoracic extension mobility (p. 73)

▶ **Heart disease.** Symptoms of heart disease increase with physical exertion that raises the pulse rate or the blood pressure, such as climbing the stairs. Movements of the thoracic spine, on the other hand, have little or no effect on these symptoms.

The symptoms of heart disease can vary greatly. Symptoms such as tachycardia, shortness of breath, cold sweats, or nausea may or may not be present. A classic symptom is a feeling of pressure and tightness in the chest, sometimes also radiating to the left arm or jaw. Women especially may experience a diffuse back or stomach pain instead.

Exertion-induced symptoms

The increase of symptoms with cardiovascular exertion is a more reliable indication of heart disease than is the type of symptom a patient reports. If there is any doubt, the patient should always be examined by a cardiologist.

Shortness of breath can also be the result of a lung disease. Possible signs of lung disease are:
- Breath sounds that are audible without a stethoscope or placing an ear on the patient's chest
- Enlarged, convex fingernails
- Thickening of the distal phalanges
- A hypomobile thorax fixed in an inspiratory position
- Chest breathing
- Hypertrophic accessory inspiration musculature

Biomechanics

Endurance sports with smooth, cyclical movements promote spinal fitness in many ways:
- Rigid myofascial holding patterns and muscular imbalances are resolved.
- Coordination improves.
- The metabolism of all the tissues is stimulated.
- Strength and endurance of the postural muscles is improved.
- The patient's mood is improved, which in many studies has been found to be an important requirement for a healthy spine.

Warm-up stretching

Mobility exercises are helpful immediately before and after endurance training, but they are particularly important before endurance training because the joints are optimally tuned up by mobility exercises, before being loaded by activities such as jogging. While this does not prevent acute injuries, it does make movement during the endurance training smoother and prevents degenerative joint wear.

Alternative Tests and Exercises for Groups and When the Floor or Wall Cannot be Used

10 Alternative Tests and Exercises for Groups and When the Floor or Wall Cannot be Used

This chapter contains alternative tests and exercises for groups (p. 130) and for situations in which the tests and exercises must be performed without the possibility of lying down (p. 127), kneeling (p. 132), or exclusively at the participants' seats (p. 136). These are summarized in **Table 10.1** with the following table cell entries:

Tests that are marked with "Q & A" (question and answer) require only a verbal response, whereas tests that are marked "Demo plus Q & A" require a demonstration by the therapist of the correct procedure, followed by a verbal response from the patient. Moreover, "not possible" refers to tests which cannot be done in the respective situation, the inserted page references refer to the respective alternative test or exercise, and blank cells refer to situations where no alternative is required because the original versions of the tests described in Chapters 3 to 9 can be used.

Original exercises

The original exercises are more precisely targeted and effective than the alternatives. Therefore, wherever the situation permits, the original exercises should be preferred over the alternative exercises.

Tab. 10.1 Alternative tests and exercises

	Individual treatment	Groups	Without kneeling or lying down	Seated
Posture (12 tests)				
Seated posture with symmetrical foot placement				
Neutral spinal curvature				
Sitting without side bending or twisting				
Stabilized neutral spinal curvature				
Balanced upper body				
Posture-friendly environment	Q & A	Q & A	Q & A	Q & A
Chair height				
Distance between the knees and between the feet				
Symmetrical weight distribution when sitting				
Stance width				
Symmetrical weight distribution when standing				
Standing posture with a balanced upper body				
Relaxation (5 tests)				
Relaxed tongue				
Relaxed lower jaw				
Relaxed lower lip				
Relaxed shoulders				
Abdominal breathing				
Movement (3 tests)				
Changing seated position	Q & A	Q & A	Q & A	Q & A
Change of position	Q & A	Q & A	Q & A	Q & A
Dynamic sitting and standing				

Tab. 10.1 Alternative tests and exercises *(continued)*

	Individual treatment	Groups	Without kneeling or lying down	Seated
Coordination (5 tests)				
Sitting up		Demo plus Q & A	Demo plus Q & A	Demo plus Q & A
Balance				
Arm swing				Not possible
Hip extension				Not possible
Eye muscle coordination				
Mobility (16 tests)				
Chin tuck mobility				p. 72 (**Fig. 7.5**)
Thoracic extension mobility				Not possible
Back muscle flexibility			p. 132	p. 132
Shoulder mobility			p. 132	p. 136
Finger flexor flexibility				p. 137
Arm nerve mobility		p. 83		Not possible
Rotational mobility			p. 133	p. 137
Lifting technique				
Hip flexion mobility				p. 138
Buttock muscle flexibility				p. 138
Leg, back, and cranial nerve mobility				p. 139
Posterior thigh flexibility		p. 130	p. 133	p. 133
Calf flexibility				p. 139
Inner thigh flexibility		Not possible	Not possible	Not possible
Hip extension mobility		p. 131		p. 140
Anterior thigh flexibility			p. 133	p. 133
Strength (3 tests)				
Abdominal and anterior neck muscle strength			p. 134	p. 134
Back muscle strength			Not possible	Not possible
Shoulder blade and triceps muscle strength				p. 140
Endurance (1 test)				
Endurance: minutes per week	Q & A	Q & A	Q & A	Q & A

10.1 Alternative Tests and Exercises for Groups

Rooms for group work usually do not have enough corners and door frames to simultaneously test all the participants in a group for posterior thigh flexibility (p. 101) or hip extension mobility (p. 109). To allow for the simultaneous testing of all group members, the following alternatives may be used.

10.1.1 Posterior Thigh Flexibility

▶ **Starting position.** Lie on your back so that your left buttock (**Fig. 10.1**, ①) touches the leg of a standing helper. Place a pillow under your head if you cannot pass the chin tuck mobility and thoracic extension mobility tests (pp. 70 and 73).

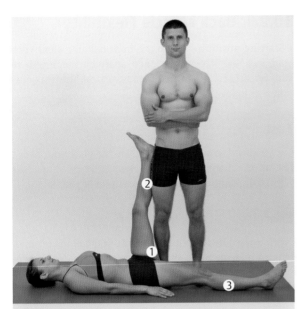

Fig. 10.1 Alternative exercise with a helper instead of a door frame.

Test

Without experiencing tension or pain, can you push your heel so far up on the helper's leg (and thus stretch your left leg so far) that your left calf touches the helper (Fig. **10.1**, ②) while your right leg lies so flat on the floor that your right calf touches the floor (Fig. **10.1**, ③)?

Exercise

Extend your left knee until you feel the onset of tension. Remain in this position until the tension resolves. The helper remains standing in the same position the whole time and does not change the position of your left leg. Only you will determine the amount of knee extension and how much tension you would like to generate.

10.1.2 Hip Extension Mobility

▶ **Starting position.** Stand with your back against a wall. One hand should lie flat between the sacrum and the wall, so that the inner surface of your hand touches the wall, while your thumb lies at the middle of your waistband and your fingers lie below the waistband (**Fig. 10.2**).Your left foot should be placed with the heel against the wall and your toes pointing straight forward. Your right foot should then be placed flat on a stool or a chair that is positioned one step forward. If you are not wearing a bra, imagine you were. Push your lower back toward the wall, until your real or imaginary bra strap (**Fig. 10.2**, ①) is in firm contact with the wall (**Fig. 10.3**, ②).

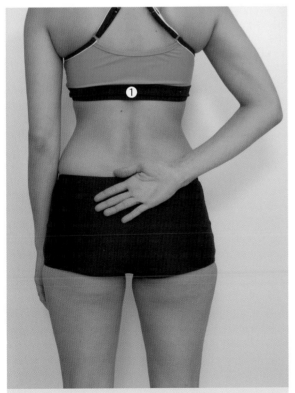

Fig. 10.2 One hand between the sacrum and the wall ...

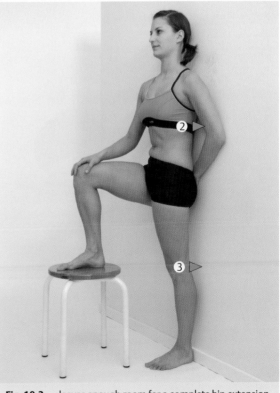

Fig. 10.3 ... leaves enough room for a complete hip extension.

Test

Can you maintain this contact without pain or tension in your left groin or hip while you extend your left knee completely (**Fig. 10.3**, ③)?

Exercise

Work toward the test objective until you feel a stop and/or the onset of tension in your groin or hip and maintain this position until you can go further and/or the tension lessens.

10.2 Alternative Tests and Exercises without Lying Down

These alternatives are suitable for situations in which kneeling or lying on the floor is not an option. Examples are when the floor is dirty and mats are not available, or where there is not enough space to exercise on the floor. These alternatives are also helpful when working with older persons who can no longer get down to or up from the floor.

10.2.1 Back Muscle Flexibility

▶ **Starting position.** Sit on the front half of a chair with your feet and knees positioned apart by the length of your forearm (p. 29) and your shins vertical. The test question is as follows.

Test

Can you bend so far forward that you can place your hands flat on the floor and see the underside of your chair (**Fig. 10.4**), without experiencing tension or pain?

Exercise

Work toward the test objective until you feel the onset of tension and maintain this position until the tension resolves.

10.2.2 Shoulder Mobility

The alternative shoulder mobility test and exercise differ from the original (p. 78) only in that they are done with the back leaning against a wall (**Fig. 10.5**) rather than with the patient lying down (p. 78).

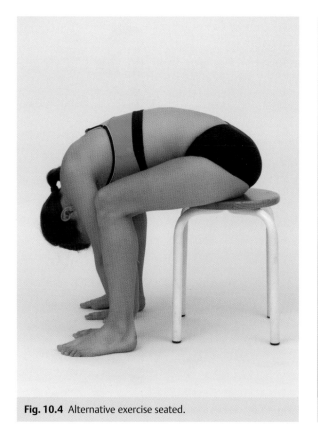

Fig. 10.4 Alternative exercise seated.

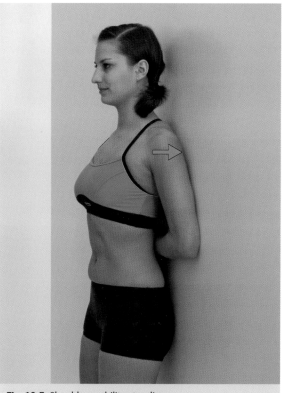

Fig. 10.5 Shoulder mobility standing.

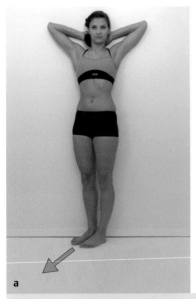
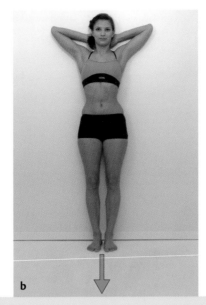
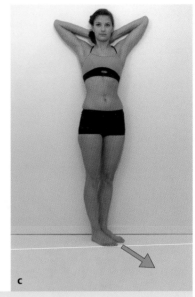

Fig. 10.6 Rotational mobility standing.

10.2.3 Rotational Mobility

▶ **Starting position.** Stand with your back against a wall and place your feet far enough from the wall that your legs are vertical (**Fig. 10.6a–c**). Lock your fingers behind your neck and touch the wall with both your elbows. Tip your head so far forward that you can see the front of your body (feet, chest, or abdomen) and hold this "double chin" position, while you push your neck toward the wall until one finger touches the wall. Imagine that your feet are standing at the 12 o'clock position on a clock dial (**Fig. 10.6b**).

Test

Can you leave your finger and both elbows in contact with the wall while you place your feet first on the 2 o'clock (**Fig. 10.6a**) and then on the 10 o'clock position (**Fig. 10.6c**), without experiencing any tension or pain?

Exercise

Work toward the test objective until you feel the onset of tension and maintain this position until the tension resolves.

10.2.4 Posterior Thigh Flexibility

▶ **Starting position.** Sit on the front edge of a chair with your spine in neutral curvature (p. 12). Stretch your left leg forward and relax your left foot. Press both elbows against your sides. Lean forward from the hips with an undiminished lumbar arch and your elbows locked against your sides.

Test

Can you lean forward until your fingers reach both kneecaps (**Fig. 10.7**), without experiencing tension or pain?

Exercise

Work toward the test objective until you feel the onset of tension and maintain this position until the tension resolves.

10.2.5 Anterior Thigh Flexibility

▶ **Starting position.** Stand up from a chair with arms and turn one quarter turn to the left. You should only pick a chair with casters if your balance is good enough to do the following exercise without risk of falling. If in doubt, use a chair without casters. Then place the back of your left foot on the arm rest behind you and kneel on the seat with your left knee. Your right leg should remain on the floor. Now tip your pelvis as far as possible in the direction in which your lower back is pushed backward, while your pubic bone moves forward.

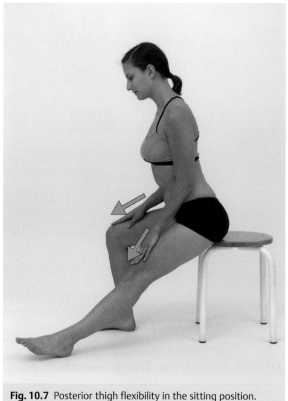

Fig. 10.7 Posterior thigh flexibility in the sitting position.

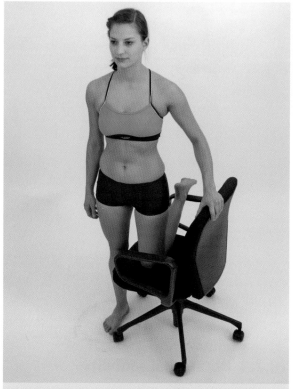

Fig. 10.8 Anterior thigh flexibility in the standing position.

Test

Can you maintain this pelvic tilt and shift your weight forward until your left thigh is vertical (**Fig. 10.8**), without experiencing pain or tension in the front of your left thigh?

Exercise

Work toward the test objective until you feel the onset of tension and maintain this position until the tension resolves.

10.2.6 Abdominal and Anterior Neck Muscle Strength

A reliable test of abdominal and anterior neck muscle strength is only possible in the supine position. These muscles may, however, also be strengthened in a seated position. For this purpose, modify the exercises for dynamic sitting and standing (p. 53) as follows.

Exercise

Lean back: Swing your upper body with a stabilized neutral spinal curvature (p. 23) back and forth between the vertical (**Fig. 10.9 a**) and the backward-leaning upper body position (**Fig. 10.9b**). Exhale when leaning backward, hold this position for 3 seconds, and inhale when returning to the vertical position.

This exercise strengthens both the abdominal and the anterior neck muscles, whereas the next two variations of the exercise train only the abdominal muscles.

Push knee forward: Push your left and right knees forward alternately (**Fig. 10.10**) without moving your chest. At the end of the movement, hold the position for 3 seconds.

Hip hike: Raise your left and right hip alternately (**Fig. 10.11**) without letting your chest move. At the end of the movement, hold the position for 3 seconds.

▶ **Exercise.** Alternate among the three variants of the exercise and repeat them until your muscles start to feel tired.

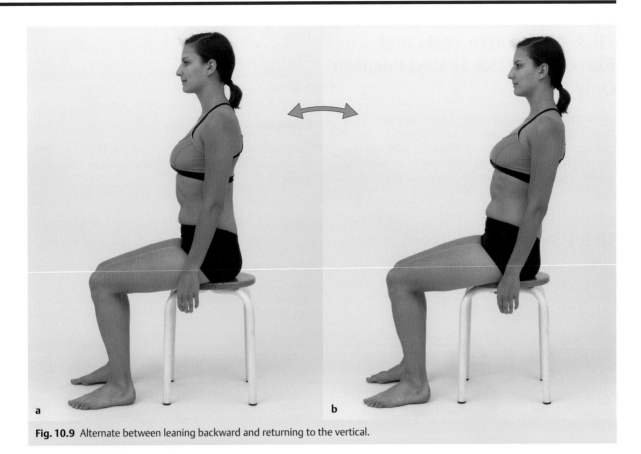

Fig. 10.9 Alternate between leaning backward and returning to the vertical.

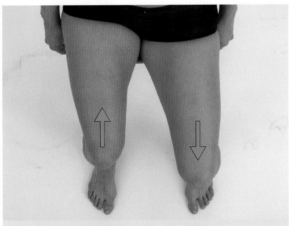

Fig. 10.10 Alternate pushing your left and right knee forward without moving your chest.

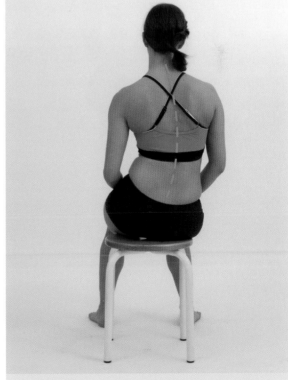

Fig. 10.11 Alternate raising your left and right hip without moving your chest.

10.3 Alternative Tests and Exercises, in the Seated Position Only

The alternative exercises to be done seated only are intended for situations in which exercise and testing will take place exclusively at a seat without a wall. For example, you may have so many participants on chairs that there is not enough space for exercises on the floor or at the wall.

10.3.1 Shoulder Mobility

▸ **Starting position.** Place your left hand at your back and slide it upward until you are touching your right shoulder blade.

Test

Can you stick your chest out while pulling your left shoulder backward (**Fig. 10.12**), without experiencing tension or pain?

Exercise

Work toward the test objective until you feel the onset of tension and maintain this position until the tension resolves.

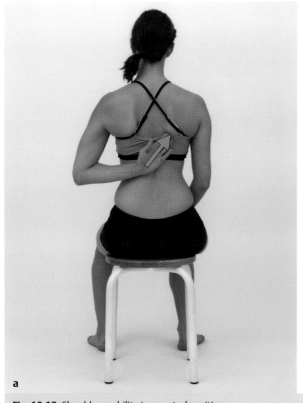
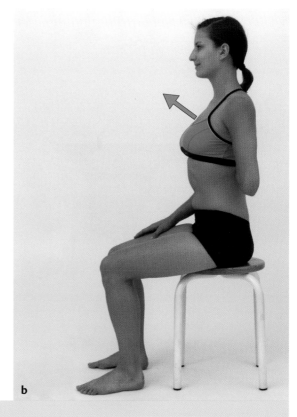
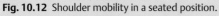

Fig. 10.12 Shoulder mobility in a seated position.

10.3.2 Finger Flexor Flexibility

▶ **Starting position.** Extend your left arm forward horizontally and turn it outward until the inside of your wrist points upward and your elbow points downward. Then angle your wrist so that your fingers are pointing downward and the palm of your hand is pointing forward.

Test

Can you pull the fingers of your left hand toward you with your right hand until the fingers of the left hand point vertically downward (**Fig. 10.13**), without experiencing pain or tension?

Exercise

Work toward the test objective until you feel the onset of tension and maintain this position until the tension resolves.

10.3.3 Rotational Mobility

▶ **Starting position.** For rotational mobility (**Fig. 10.14 a–c**), sit with your upper body erect (sticking your chest out). Lock your fingers at your neck and pull your elbows back until they point to the sides in opposite directions (**Fig. 10.14 b**).

Test

Can you turn your upper body an eighth of a turn to the left (**Fig. 10.14 a**) and to the right (**Fig. 10.14 c**), without experiencing pain or tension?

Exercise

Work toward the test objective until you feel the onset of tension and maintain this position until the tension resolves.

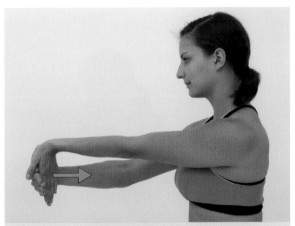

Fig. 10.13 Finger flexor flexibility in a seated position.

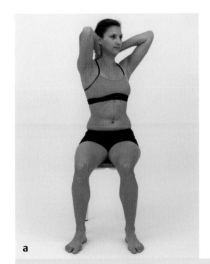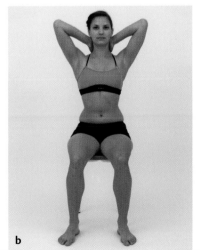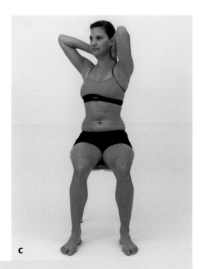

a   b   c

Fig. 10.14 Rotational mobility in a seated position.

10.3.4 Hip Flexion Mobility

▶ **Starting position.** Sit with your spine 75% erect (see **Fig. 3.4**) and feel how far your lumbar spine is arched in this position. Press your elbows to your body at the sides, and place your hands flat on your thighs. Lean forward from the hips with an undiminished lumbar arch and your elbows still locked against your sides.

Test

Can you lean forward until your fingers reach the lower edge of both kneecaps (**Fig. 10.15**), without experiencing tension or pain?

Exercise

Work toward the test objective until you feel the onset of tension and maintain this position until the tension resolves.

10.3.5 Buttock Muscle Flexibility

▶ **Starting position.** Sit with your spine 75% erect (see **Fig. 3.4**) and feel how far your lumbar spine is arched in this position. Then place your left foot on your right thigh, return your lumbar spine to 75% arching, and press your elbows locked against your sides. Lean forward from the hips with an undiminished lumbar arch and your elbows still locked against your trunk.

Test

Can you lean forward until the fingers of both hands reach your left shin (**Fig. 10.16**), without experiencing tension or pain?

Exercise

Work toward the test objective until you feel the onset of tension and maintain this position until the tension resolves.

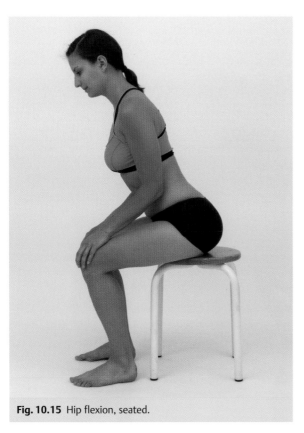

Fig. 10.15 Hip flexion, seated.

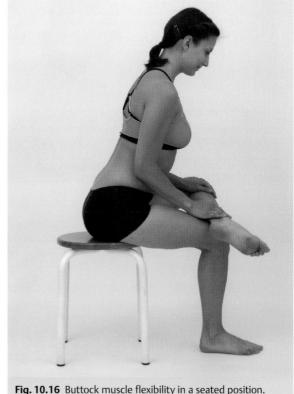

Fig. 10.16 Buttock muscle flexibility in a seated position.

10.3.6 Leg, Back, and Cranial Nerve Mobility

▸ **Starting position.** Sit at the front edge of a chair with your shins vertical. Place your knees apart by the length of a forearm (see **Fig. 3.23**). Advance your left foot by one foot length, actively pull your left foot up toward your left knee as far as possible, and keep it there.

Test

Can you bend forward until you can see the underside of your chair (**Fig. 10.17**), without experiencing tension or pain?

Exercise

Work toward the test objective until you feel the onset of tension and maintain this position until the tension resolves.

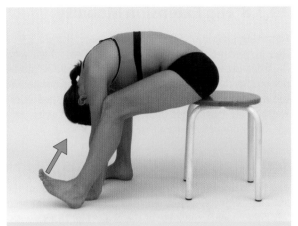

Fig. 10.17 Leg, back, and cranial nerve mobility in a seated position.

10.3.7 Calf Flexibility

▸ **Starting position.** Sit on the front edge of a chair and lean against the wall. Extend your left knee completely, with your left heel resting on the floor.

Test

Can you pull your left foot toward your left knee until the sole of your shoe or foot is vertical, without experiencing tension or pain?

Exercise

Work toward the test objective until you feel the onset of tension and maintain this position until the tension resolves (**Fig. 10.18**).

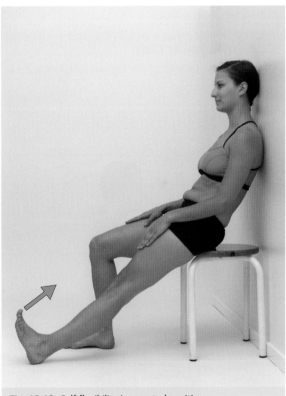

Fig. 10.18 Calf flexibility in a seated position.

10.3.8 Hip Extension Mobility

► **Starting position.** Stand facing the side of a chair. The toes of your left foot should be on the floor, flush with the front edge of the chair. Your right foot should be placed flat on the chair seat. Tip your pelvis as far as possible in the direction in which your lower back is pushed backward, while your pubic bone moves forward. Keep your left knee completely extended.

Test

Can you maintain this pelvic tilt and the extension of the left knee, while you shift your weight forward, until your left knee touches the edge of the chair (**Fig. 10.19**), without experiencing tension or pain in your left groin or hip?

Exercise

Work toward the test objective until you feel the onset of tension in your left hip or groin and maintain this position until the tension resolves.

> **Caution: Runaway chair**
>
> At work, you should not do this exercise with a desk chair with casters because it could roll away.

10.3.9 Shoulder Blade and Triceps Muscle Strength

► **Starting position.** Sit on a chair, with two hand widths between your buttocks and the back rest. Then press your elbows so hard against the back rest that your back is pushed away from the back rest completely and as far as possible (**Fig. 10.20**).

Test

Can you hold this position (**Fig. 10.20**) without trembling, pain, or considerable effort for 60 seconds?

Exercise

Hold this position until you feel your muscles tiring.

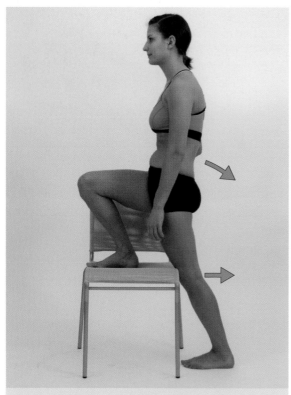

Fig. 10.19 Hip extension mobility without a wall.

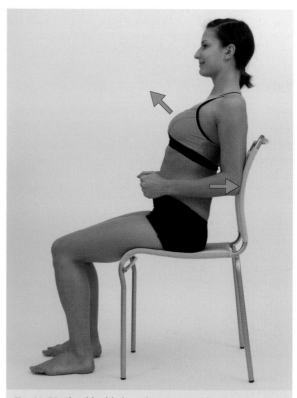

Fig. 10.20 Shoulder blade and triceps muscle strength in a seated position.

Manual Techniques
and Helpful Tools

11 Manual Techniques

Most spine problems can be treated effectively, gently, and with a lasting effect using the exercise system presented in this book.

For instance, the correction of twisted vertebrae using the exercises in this book is often more efficacious and long-lasting than with manual techniques. The right exercises for repositioning specific vertebrae are described in Navigator 26 (p. 177).

In case, however, correct performance of the mobility exercises does not result in improved mobility, the related "Troubleshooting" sections suggest alternative exercises, and in some cases manual techniques, that can facilitate progress toward the mobility test goals. These manual techniques are described on the following pages.

With all the techniques, the procedure is as follows. The patient lies supine on a treatment table. The therapist exerts a gentle, continuous pressure on the tissue under examination. If the tissue yields easily, there is no need for treatment. If the resistance is strong, the therapist goes as far as the first resistance, maintains a steady pressure, and at the same time guides the patient verbally through the individual exercises given in Chapter 4, on "Relaxation" (pp. 39–49) until the tension in the tissue decreases perceptibly.

If the tension always eases during a particular relaxation exercise, the key to relaxation has been found. The patient is then asked to focus on this particular relaxation exercise throughout her daily activities. Thus, the primary objective of the manual pressure is to help the patient feel and deliberately release tensions of which she had not been aware.

Autogenic mobilization

The patient effects the mobilization with the key relaxation exercise you have helped her to discover. The gentle pressure of your fingers merely serves to focus the patient on the relevant area, and allows you to provide her with feedback once she manages to relax. If you use manual techniques to solve blockades in this manner, you will be achieving lasting results while preventing premature arthritis in your own finger joints.

As with all the tests and exercises, the following manual techniques are contraindicated if they produce effects that go beyond normal sensitivity to pressure and cause pain.

11.1 First Rib

The therapist sits at the patient's head, makes contact with the dorsal aspect of the first rib on each side, and pushes it in an anterior direction (**Fig. 11.1**).

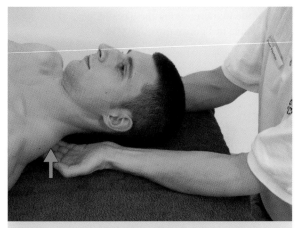

Fig. 11.1 Manual mobilization of the first rib.

11.2 Left Glenohumeral Joint

The therapist stands at the patient's left side. The patient's hands rest on his abdomen.

The therapist's right hand stabilizes the patient's scapula by grasping its medial edge with the fingers, while the thenar eminence supports the spine of the scapula. The fingers at the edge of the scapula prevent the scapula from gliding off in a medial direction. The thenar eminence prevents dorsal movement of the scapula.

With the fingers of his left hand, the therapist slides the head of the humerus along the glenoid fossa of the stabilized scapula in a dorsal direction (**Fig. 11.2**).

11.3 Left Pectoralis Minor

The therapist stands at the patient's left side facing the pectoralis minor. The index and middle fingers of one hand hook into the cranial edge of pectoralis minor, directly medial to the coracoid process. The therapist supports the index and middle finger of one hand with the fingers of the other hand, and pulls the muscle perpendicular to the grain of the muscle fibers in a caudal, lateral, and slightly dorsal direction (**Fig. 11.3**).

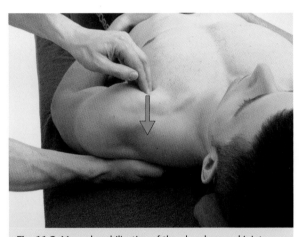

Fig. 11.2 Manual mobilization of the glenohumeral joint.

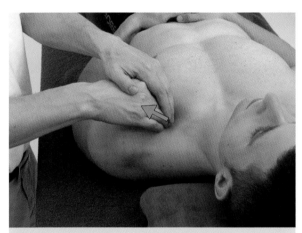

Fig. 11.3 Manual release of the pectoralis minor.

11.4 Psoas and Iliacus

11.4.1 Contraindications

> **Contraindications**
>
> Manual pressure on the psoas and iliacus is absolutely contraindicated in pregnancy, aortic aneurysm, and all postoperative conditions, tumors, or inflammatory diseases of the abdominal cavity.

Specific examples of inflammatory diseases of the abdominal cavity are appendicitis, Crohn disease, and diverticulitis. Pressure must also not be exerted on the abdomen if an arterial pulse can be felt under the fingers. The contraindications to the technique must always be explained to the patient before beginning. On first use of this technique, in addition to obtaining the patient's explicit permission, the therapist must ask: "Is there any reason why I should not apply pressure to your abdomen?"

11.4.2 Left Psoas

The patient lies supine with his legs supported in hip and knee flexion. The therapist stands at the patient's left side. At a point somewhat lateral and caudal to the umbilicus, the therapist slowly and carefully lets his fingers sink into the abdominal wall, in a dorsal direction, until they contact the psoas. Then the fingers engage the psoas by gently pushing its muscle belly in a dorsolateral direction (**Fig. 11.4**).

11.4.3 Left Iliacus

The patient lies supine with his legs supported in hip and knee flexion. The therapist stands at the patient's left side and contacts the iliac crest about three finger widths dor-

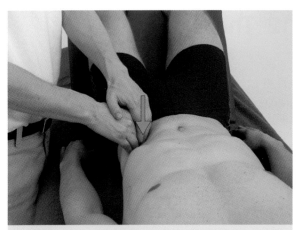

Fig. 11.5 Manual release of the iliacus.

sal to the anterior superior iliac spine in order to avoid the inguinal ligament. Starting at this point, the therapist allows his fingers to sink in slowly and carefully along the medial surface of the ilium in a dorsal direction until they engage the iliacus (**Fig. 11.5**).

11.5 Talocrural Joint

The patient lies supine on the treatment table with his heels hanging over the foot end of the table. The therapist stands at the foot end of the table facing the patient. The therapist supports the patient's heel against the left side of his groin and uses his abdomen to bring the patient' talocrural joint into dorsiflexion until he feels the first slight resistance. One of the therapist's hands cups and stabilizes the ankle mortise from the dorsal side, while at the same time the other hand slides the talus along the malleoli in a dorsal direction (**Fig. 11.6**).

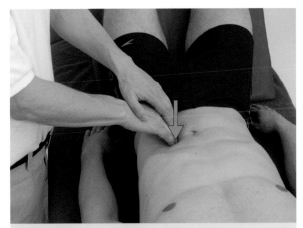

Fig. 11.4 Manual release of the psoas muscle.

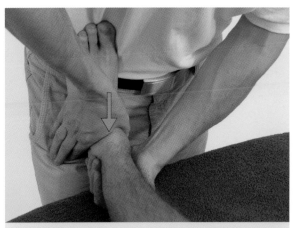

Fig. 11.6 Manual mobilization of the talocrural joint.

12 The Navigator

▶ **Body diagram.** On the body diagram (**Fig. 12.1**), select the part of the body where your patient's symptom or dysfunction is located. There you will find a Navigator chart number. On the corresponding chart, there is a list of possible causes of the symptom or dysfunction with suggestions for appropriate tests and exercises. This list is sorted by relevance, starting with the cause that is most often responsible for problems in the respective area, along with the matching test and exercise to identify and solve it.

▶ **Background color.** In addition to the order, the likelihood by which a test and exercise may detect and solve

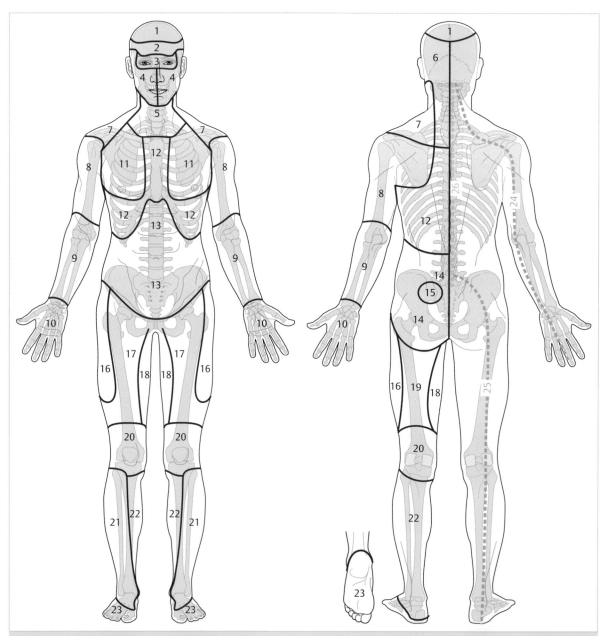

Fig. 12.1 Body diagram for the Navigator charts. The numbers indicate the Navigator chart that contains the appropriate tests and exercises for the evaluation and treatment of symptoms and dysfunctions in the respective region.

the underlying cause of a problem in a particular area is indicated by its background color. The tests and exercises that most frequently lead to resolution of the symptom or dysfunction in the particular body area have a dark orange background. Tests and exercises that less frequently lead to a solution have a light orange background.

▶ **Procedure.** If the first exercise leads to the desired result, no further steps are necessary—simply stay with that exercise as long as it is efficacious. If the first exercise does not lead to improvement or further improvement, go on to the second exercise. If that exercise is also not efficacious, move ahead to the next exercise on the list until progress toward the treatment goal is made.

Instead of working your way down the list of exercises in order, you may of course also start with an exercise further down the list if the signs, your experience, or other information leads you to believe that the cause that particular exercise addresses is the primary one.

▶ **Example.** (Table 12.1) Your patient has symptoms in the area at the top of her head. In the body diagram, this location is marked 1. Therefore, Navigator number 1 (p. 148) contains the relevant tests and exercises for this area.

You can see that restricted dural neurodynamics is at the top of the list in the chart and is thus ranked as the most frequent cause of cranial symptoms. Check whether this applies to your patient using the leg, back, and cranial nerve mobility test. If the test is positive, have the patient train with the leg, back, and cranial nerve mobility exercise. If the symptoms improve with this practice, you have found the solution. If not, the next step is to check whether your patient slouches while sitting. If you observe, however, that your patient is not slouching, but tends toward marked chest breathing, you can omit all the exercises from "Neutral spinal" curvature to "Relaxed lower lip" and start with "Abdominal breathing."

Table 12.1   Example of a navigator chart

Navigator 1—Top of the Head

Possible functional causes of symptoms or dysfunctions	Tests and exercises
Restricted dural neurodynamics	Leg, back, and cranial nerve mobility (p. 98)
Slouching while sitting	Neutral spinal curvature (p. 12)
Hypertonic jaw muscles	Relaxed lower jaw (p. 41)
The tongue is habitually pushed so far to the front or the side that it touches the teeth	Relaxed tongue (p. 39)
The lower lip is habitually pushed upward	Relaxed lower lip (p. 43)
Chest breathing	Abdominal breathing (p. 47)
The shoulders are raised or protracted	Relaxed shoulders (p. 45)
Excessive and hypomobile thoracic spine kyphosis	Thoracic extension mobility (p. 73)

Navigator 1—Top of the Head

Possible functional causes of symptoms or dysfunctions	Tests and exercises
Restricted dural neurodynamics	Leg, back, and cranial nerve mobility (p. 98)
Slouching while sitting	Neutral spinal curvature (p. 12)
Hypertonic jaw muscles	Relaxed lower jaw (p. 41)
The tongue is habitually pushed so far to the front or the side that it touches the teeth	Relaxed tongue (p. 39)
Lower lip habitually pushed upward	Relaxed lower lip (p. 43)
Chest breathing	Abdominal breathing (p. 47)
Shoulders are raised or protracted	Relaxed shoulders (p. 45)
Excessive and hypomobile thoracic spine kyphosis	Thoracic extension mobility (p. 73)

Navigator 2—Forehead

Possible functional causes of symptoms or dysfunctions	Tests and exercises
Dysfunction of the atlantooccipital joint, jaw muscles, or occipitofrontalis because of cervical spine hyperextension to compensate for a thoracic extension deficit	Thoracic extension mobility (p. 73)
Dysfunction of the cervical spine, occipitofrontalis, eyes, and jaw resulting from shortened neck extensors	Chin tuck mobility (p. 70)
Cranial tension and muscle guarding resulting from restricted dural neurodynamics	Leg, back, and cranial nerve mobility (p. 98)
Dysfunction of the cervical spine, occipitofrontalis, eyes, and the jaw resulting from a habitual forward head position	Neutral spinal curvature (p. 12)
Hypertonic masseter, temporalis, medial pterygoid, or lateral pterygoid due to keeping the jaw tight	Relaxed lower jaw (p. 41)
Hypertonic masseter, temporalis, and medial pterygoid due to chest breathing	Abdominal breathing (p. 47)
Hypertonic lateral pterygoid, anterior portions of temporalis, or masseter resulting from a habit of contacting the teeth with the tongue	Relaxed tongue (p. 39)
Synergistic hypertonicity of the lateral pterygoid, anterior portions of temporalis, and masseter in order to keep the lower lip raised	Relaxed lower lip (p. 43)
Synergistic hypertonicity of the masseter, temporalis, and medial pterygoid muscles due to a holding pattern of the upper trapezius muscles	Relaxed shoulders (p. 45)
Frontal headaches caused by an imbalance of the eye muscles	Eye muscle coordination (p. 65)

Navigator 3—Eyes

Potential functional causes of symptoms or dysfunctions	Tests and exercises
Dysfunction of the atlantooccipital joint caused by sitting with a forward head	Neutral spinal curvature (p. 12)
Dysfunction of the atlantooccipital joint caused by cervical hyperextension that compensates for a lack of thoracic extension mobility	Thoracic extension mobility (p. 73)
Tense eye muscles	Eye muscle coordination (p. 65)
Tension in the lateral pterygoid and thus pull at its origin, the sphenoid bone, to counteract the posterior reaction force of the incisors when the tongue presses against the incisors	Relaxed tongue (p. 39)
Tightness of the masseter, temporalis, medial pterygoid, or lateral pterygoid due to keeping the jaw tight	Relaxed lower jaw (p. 41)
Synergistic hypertonicity of the lateral pterygoid, anterior portions of temporalis, or masseter muscles when the lower lip is raised habitually	Relaxed lower lip (p. 43)
Synergistic tightness of the masseter, temporalis, and medial pterygoid with a holding pattern of the upper trapezius muscles	Relaxed shoulders (p. 45)
Synergistic tightness of the masseter, temporalis, and medial pterygoid with chest breathing	Abdominal breathing (p. 47)
Dysfunction of cervical spine, eyes, and jaw due to a habitual forward head posture	Chin tuck mobility (p. 70)

Navigator 4—Jaw and Temples

Potential functional causes of symptoms or dysfunctions	Tests and exercises
Hypertonic masseter, temporalis, medial pterygoid, or lateral pterygoid due to a habit of protruding the jaw and/or keeping it tight	Relaxed lower jaw (p. 41)
Tension in the lateral pterygoid and thus pull at its origin, the sphenoid bone, to counteract the posterior reaction force of the incisors when the tongue presses against the incisors	Relaxed tongue (p. 39)
Synergistic hypertonicity of the lateral pterygoid, anterior portions of temporalis, and masseter, when the lower lip is raised	Relaxed lower lip (p. 43)
Synergistic hypertonicity of the masseter, temporalis, and medial pterygoid due to a holding pattern of the upper trapezius muscles	Relaxed shoulders (p. 45)
Synergistic hypertonicity of the masseter, temporalis, and medial pterygoid muscles with chest breathing	Abdominal breathing (p. 47)
Temporal headaches caused by tension in the ipsilateral rectus lateralis muscle	Eye muscle coordination (p. 65)
Sitting with a forward head posture	Neutral spinal curvature (p. 12)
Synergistic tension in the jaw muscles with tension in the anterior trunk muscles in order to stabilize the upper body when it is leaning too far backward	Balanced upper body when seated (p. 25)
Cervical spine hyperextension resulting from a thoracic spine extension deficit	Thoracic extension mobility (p. 73)
Hypertonic cervical spine and jaw muscles resulting from a hypomobile brachial plexus	Arm nerve mobility (p. 83)
Hypertonic neck extensors, jaw, and eye muscles due to restricted dural neurodynamics	Leg, back, and cranial nerve mobility (p. 98)
Tense cervical spine, eye, and jaw muscles resulting from a habitually static posture	Dynamic sitting and standing (p. 53)
Dysfunction of the cervical spine, eyes, and jaw due to a habitual forward head posture	Chin tuck mobility (p. 70)
Temporomandibular tightness and joint dysfunction resulting from an anterior pelvic shift	Standing posture with a balanced upper body (p. 36)

Navigator 5—Ventral Neck

Potential functional causes of symptoms or dysfunctions	Tests and exercises
Overstretched ventral neck muscles and fascia due to a forward head posture	Neutral spinal curvature (p. 12)
Synergistic tension in the supra- and infrahyoid muscles and fascia with chest breathing	Abdominal breathing (p. 47)
Tension in the ventral neck muscles that is required to stabilize the head when the upper body is leaning too far backward	Balanced upper body when seated (p. 25)
Overstretched ventral neck muscles and fascia resulting from a forward head posture with neck retraction hypomobility	Chin tuck mobility (p. 70)
Overstretching of the supra- and infrahyoid muscles and fascia resulting from a forward head posture that compensates for a thoracic spine extension deficit	Thoracic extension mobility (p. 73)
Tension in the suprahyoid muscles to counteract the posterior reaction force of the incisors when the tongue presses against the incisors	Relaxed tongue (p. 39)
Tension in the suprahyoid and laryngeal muscles due to a habit of protruding the lower jaw	Relaxed lower jaw (p. 41)
Synergistic tension in the supra- and infrahyoid muscles and fascia due to a holding pattern of the upper trapezius muscles	Relaxed shoulders (p. 45)
Synergistic tightness of the anterior neck muscles and fascia when the lower lip is habitually raised	Relaxed lower lip (p. 43)
Ventral neck muscles hypertonicity resulting from an anterior pelvic shift	Standing posture with a balanced upper body (p. 36)
Weakness of the anterior neck muscles	Abdominal and anterior neck muscle strength (p. 117)

Navigator 6—Occiput and Dorsal Cervical Spine

Potential functional causes of symptoms or dysfunctions	Tests and exercises
Sitting with a forward head posture	Neutral spinal curvature (p. 12)
Hyperextended cervical spine resulting from a thoracic spine extension deficit	Thoracic extension mobility (p. 73)
Ergonomic factors that prevent a neutral and dynamic posture	Posture-friendly environment (p. 27)
Hypertonic shoulder elevator muscles	Relaxed shoulders (p. 45)
Shifting the head forward to compensate for a lack of hip flexion when leaning forward	Stabilized neutral spinal curvature (p. 23)
Asymmetrical stress on the spine caused by an asymmetrical spinal posture	Sitting without side bending or twisting (p. 21)
Hypertonic shoulder and neck muscles resulting from chest breathing	Abdominal breathing (p. 47)
Restricted eye movement compensated for by tightness of the neck muscles	Eye muscle coordination (p. 65)
Tension in the neck muscles caused by tension in the jaw muscles	Relaxed lower jaw (p. 41)
Tension in the neck muscles caused by a habit of pushing the tongue so far to the front or the side that it touches the teeth	Relaxed tongue (p. 39)
Synergistic tension in the anterior neck muscles and fascia when the lower lip is habitually raised	Relaxed lower lip (p. 43)
Protracted cervical spine due to a lack of retraction mobility	Chin tuck mobility (p. 70)
Hypertonic neck extensors and cervical spine hypomobility caused by restricted dural neurodynamics	Leg, back, and cranial nerve mobility (p. 98)
Static stress on the spine	Dynamic sitting and standing (p. 53)
Lack of spinal rotation in walking	Arm swing (p. 62)
Habitual shoulder protrusion resulting from a lack of internal rotation of the glenohumeral joint	Shoulder mobility (p. 78)
Stress on the cervical spine resulting from restriction of thoracic spine extension, thoracic spine rotation, pectoral flexibility, and/or neuro-dynamics of the brachial plexus	Rotational mobility (p. 90)
Hypertonic shoulder elevator and protractor muscles resulting from a hypomobile and irritable brachial plexus	Arm nerve mobility (p. 83)
Imbalance of the cervical spine muscles because the upper body is leaning too far forward or backward	Balanced upper body when seated (p. 25)
Cervical spine instability and hyperextension resulting from weak and overstretched anterior neck muscles	Abdominal and anterior neck muscle strength (p. 117)
Twisted vertebrae and insufficient thoracic extension resulting from insufficient or asymmetrical back extensor strength	Back muscle strength (p. 118)
Habitual shoulder protrusion and forward head posture because of weak scapular retractor muscles	Shoulder blade and triceps muscle strength (p. 120)
Tightness that can be resolved by repeated, cyclical, alternating, and symmetrical movements	Endurance (p. 123)
Muscular asymmetry and a nonneutral cervical spine posture resulting from an anterior pelvic shift	Standing posture with a balanced upper body (p. 36)
Asymmetrical stress on the cervical spine due to an asymmetrical weight distribution when sitting	Symmetrical weight distribution when sitting (p. 30)

Navigator 7—Lateral Aspect of the Neck

Potential functional causes of symptoms or dysfunctions	Tests and exercises
Hypertonic shoulder elevator muscles	Relaxed shoulders (p. 45)
Hypertonic shoulder and neck muscles resulting from chest breathing	Abdominal breathing (p. 47)
Sitting with a forward head	Neutral spinal curvature (p. 12)
Hypertonic shoulder elevator and protractor muscles in order to compensate for a hypomobile brachial plexus	Arm nerve mobility (p. 83)
Ergonomic factors that prevent a neutral, dynamic spine and shoulder posture	Posture-friendly environment (p. 27)
Habitual shoulder protrusion to compensate for a lack of internal rotation of the glenohumeral joint	Shoulder mobility (p. 78)
Cervical spine hyperextension resulting from a restricted thoracic spine extension	Thoracic extension mobility (p. 73)
Asymmetrical stress on the spine and shoulder caused by a posture with a twisted spine	Sitting without side bending or twisting (p. 21)
Hypertonic neck extensor and shoulder elevator muscles due to restricted neurodynamics of the dura mater	Leg, back, and cranial nerve mobility (p. 98)
Restricted eye movement compensated for by asymmetrical head posture and movement	Eye muscle coordination (p. 65)
Static holding pattern in the shoulder girdle and cervical spine muscles	Arm swing (p. 62)
Shifting the head forward to compensate for a lack of hip flexion when leaning forward	Stabilized neutral spinal curvature (p. 23)
Protracted cervical spine due to a lack of retraction mobility	Chin tuck mobility (p. 70).
Tension in the neck muscles resulting from tense jaw muscles	Relaxed lower jaw (p. 41)
Tension in the neck muscles caused by a habit of pushing the tongue so far to the front or the side that it touches the teeth	Relaxed tongue (p. 39)
Tension in the neck muscles that is associated with a habitually raised lower lip	Relaxed lower lip (p. 43)
Static loading of the spine	Dynamic sitting and standing (p. 53)
Neck tension as compensation for a lack of pectoral flexibility, neurodynamics of the brachial plexus, thoracic spine extension, and/or cervical spine rotation	Rotational mobility (p. 90)
Habitual shoulder protrusion and forward head posture caused by weak scapular retractor muscles	Shoulder blade and triceps muscle strength (p. 120)
Imbalance of the spine-stabilizing muscles because the upper body is leaning too far forward or backward	Balanced upper body when seated (p. 25)
Asymmetrical stress on the cervical spine due to an asymmetrical weight distribution while sitting	Symmetrical weight distribution when sitting (p. 30)
Protracted head and protracted shoulders due to an anterior pelvic shift	Standing posture with a balanced upper body (p. 36)

Navigator 8—Shoulder and Upper Arm

Potential functional causes of symptoms or dysfunctions	Tests and exercises
Habitual shoulder protrusion resulting from a lack of internal rotation of the glenohumeral joint	Shoulder mobility (p. 78)
Hypomobility of the brachial plexus, lack of pectoral and elbow flexor flexibility, and/or a thoracic extension deficit	Rotational mobility (p. 90)
Hypertonic shoulder elevator, shoulder protractor, and/or elbow flexor muscles as a result of a hypomobile brachial plexus	Arm nerve mobility (p. 83)
Protracted shoulders caused by a weakness of the spinal extensors and scapular retractors	Neutral spinal curvature (p. 12)
Blockade of the shoulder flexion–thoracic extension kinetic chain	Thoracic extension mobility (p. 73)
Muscular imbalance between (1) hypertonic shoulder protractor and elbow flexor muscles, and (2) weak shoulder retractor and elbow extensor muscles	Shoulder blade and triceps muscle strength (p. 120)
Thoracic hyperkyphosis due to hypertonic pectoral muscles	Back muscle strength (p. 118)
Hypertonic shoulder elevator muscles as a result of chest breathing	Abdominal breathing (p. 47)
Nerve root irritation in the area of the cervicothoracic junction as a result of a forward head posture	Chin tuck mobility (p. 70)
Ergonomic factors that prevent a neutral dynamic posture of the arm, shoulder, and spine	Posture-friendly environment (p. 27)
Hypertonic hand flexor–elbow-flexor shoulder protractor muscle chain	Finger flexor flexibility (p. 81)
Dysfunction of the brachial plexus, shoulder, and arm as a result of hypertonic shoulder elevator muscles	Relaxed shoulders (p. 45)
Tension in the shoulder and arm muscles resulting from tense jaw muscles	Relaxed lower jaw (p. 41)
Tension in the shoulder and arm muscles due to a habit of pushing the tongue so far to the front or the side that it touches the teeth	Relaxed tongue (p. 39)
Tension in the shoulder and arm that is associated with a lower lip that is habitually raised	Relaxed lower lip (p. 43)
Compensatory shoulder asymmetry caused by an asymmetrical spinal posture	Sitting without side bending or twisting (p. 21)
Static holding pattern in the shoulder and arm muscles	Arm swing (p. 62)
Asymmetrical head and shoulder posture to compensate for restricted eye movement	Eye muscle coordination (p. 65)
Tension in the shoulder and arm that can be resolved by cyclical, alternating, and symmetrical movements	Endurance (p. 123)
Forward head posture with thoracic kyphosis to compensate for a lack of hip flexion when leaning forward	Stabilized neutral spinal curvature (p. 23)
Blockade of thoracic kinetic chain mobility with shoulder movements due to a habit of keeping the upper body tilted forward or backward	Balanced upper body when seated (p. 25)
Blockade of thoracic kinetic chain mobility with shoulder movements due to a habit of keeping the pelvis shifted forward or backward	Standing posture with a balanced upper body (p. 36)
Habitual static posture	Dynamic sitting and standing (p. 53)

Navigator 9—Lower Arm

Potential functional causes of symptoms or dysfunctions	Tests and exercises
Lack of finger flexor flexibility	Finger flexor flexibility (p. 81)
Hypertonic lower arm muscles resulting from hypomobility of the brachial plexus	Arm nerve mobility (p. 83)
Hypomobility of the brachial plexus resulting from chest breathing	Abdominal breathing (p. 47)
Hypomobility of the brachial plexus resulting from hypertonic shoulder elevators	Relaxed shoulders (p. 45)
Ergonomic factors that prevent a dynamic posture or sufficient rest for the upper extremities	Posture-friendly environment (p. 27)
Nerve hypomobility and hypertonic shoulder protractor–elbow flexor–finger-flexor muscle chain	Rotational mobility (p. 90)
Tension in the upper extremity that can be resolved by cyclical, alternating, and symmetrical movements	Endurance (p. 123)
Hypertonic shoulder protractor–elbow flexor–finger flexor muscle chain	Shoulder blade and triceps muscle strength (p. 120)
Hypertonic shoulder protractor–elbow flexor–finger flexor muscle chain	Back muscle strength (p. 118)
Hypertonic shoulder protractor–elbow flexor–finger flexor muscle chain	Arm swing (p. 62)
Hypertonic shoulder protractor–elbow flexor–finger flexor muscle chain	Thoracic extension mobility (p. 73)
Habitual shoulder protraction resulting from a lack of internal rotation of the glenohumeral joint	Shoulder mobility (p. 78)
Asymmetrical posture, movement, and tension in the shoulder and arm caused by a posture with a twisted or side-bent spine	Sitting without side bending or twisting (p. 21)
Hypertonic lower arm muscles resulting from posture-related brachial plexus dysfunction	Neutral spinal curvature (p. 12)
Hypertonic lower arm muscles resulting from tense jaw muscles	Relaxed lower jaw (p. 41)
Tension in the lower arm muscles caused by a habit of pushing the tongue so far to the front or the side that it touches the teeth	Relaxed tongue (p. 39)
Tension in the lower arm muscles that is associated with a lower lip that is habitually elevated	Relaxed lower lip (p. 43)
Habitually static posture	Dynamic sitting and standing (p. 53)
Hypertonic lower arm muscles resulting from dysfunction of the brachial plexus as a result of cervical spine hyperextension while leaning forward	Stabilized neutral spinal curvature (p. 23)
Hypertonic lower arm muscles resulting from restricted dural neurodynamics	Leg, back, and cranial nerve mobility (p. 98)
Asymmetrical stress on the cervical spine due to an asymmetrical weight distribution while sitting	Symmetrical weight distribution when sitting (p. 30)

Navigator 10—Hand

Potential functional causes of symptoms or dysfunctions	Tests and exercises
Lack of finger flexor flexibility	Finger flexor flexibility (p. 81)
Irritation of spinal nerves C6–T1caused by chest breathing	Abdominal breathing (p. 47)
Irritation of the hand nerves or muscles resulting from a hypomobile brachial plexus	Arm nerve mobility (p. 83)
Prolonged repetitive hand activity in a nonneutral position of the wrist and fingers	Posture-friendly environment (p. 27)
Long periods of pressure on the ulnar sulcus, Guyon canal, or carpal tunnel	
Foraminal C6–T1 nerve root irritation caused by a nonneutral posture of the cervicothoracic junction	Neutral spinal curvature (p. 12)
Finger flexor hypertonicity	Shoulder blade and triceps muscle strength (p. 120)
Finger flexor hypertonicity	Rotational mobility (p. 90)
Finger flexor hypertonicity	Back muscle strength (p. 118)
Foraminal C6–T1 nerve root irritation caused by a nonneutral cervical spine posture	Chin tuck mobility (p. 70)
Foraminal C6–T1 nerve root irritation caused by cervical hyperextension to compensate for a thoracic extension deficit	Thoracic extension mobility (p. 73)
C6–T1 nerve irritation in the foramina or the thoracic outlet caused by hypertonic shoulder elevator muscles	Relaxed shoulders (p. 45)
C6–T1 nerve irritation caused by shoulder protrusion as compensation for a lack of internal rotation of the glenohumeral joint	Shoulder mobility (p. 78)
C6–T1 nerve irritation in the foramina or the thoracic outlet caused by an asymmetrical spinal posture	Sitting without side bending or twisting (p. 21)
Tension in the shoulder, arm, and hand muscles that can be resolved by allowing the arms to swing	Arm swing (p. 62)
Tension in the shoulder, arm, and hand that can be resolved by cyclical, alternating, and symmetrical movements	Endurance (p. 123)
Habitual static posture	Dynamic sitting and standing (p. 53)
C6–T1 nerve irritation due to tension in the neck muscles resulting from tense jaw muscles	Relaxed lower jaw (p. 41)
C6–T1 nerve irritation due to synergistic tension in the neck muscles when the tongue presses against the teeth	Relaxed tongue (p. 39)
C6–T1 nerve irritation due to tension in the neck muscles to compensate for restricted eye movement	Eye muscle coordination (p. 65)
C6–T1 nerve irritation due to tension in the neck muscles that results from a habitually raised lower lip	Relaxed lower lip (p. 43)

Navigator 11—Chest Muscles

Potential functional causes of symptoms or dysfunctions	Tests and exercises
Shoulder protraction, nerve hypomobility, and a thoracic spine extension deficit resulting from a lack of flexibility of pectoralis major and pectoralis minor	Rotational mobility (p. 90)
Nerve irritation and hypertonic shoulder elevator and protractor muscles resulting from a hypomobile brachial plexus	Arm nerve mobility (p. 83)
Costosternal syndrome and pectoral slack caused by sitting with a flexed thoracic spine	Neutral spinal curvature (p. 12)
Costosternal syndrome and tightness of the pectoral muscles resulting from a thoracic extension deficit	Thoracic extension mobility (p. 73)
Habitual shoulder protrusion resulting from weak shoulder retractors	Shoulder blade and triceps muscle strength (p. 120)
Habitual shoulder protrusion as compensation for a lack of internal rotation of the glenohumeral joint	Shoulder mobility (p. 78)
Hypertonic pectoral abdominal muscle chain	Back muscle strength (p. 118)
Hypertonic intercostal muscles resulting from chest breathing	Abdominal breathing (p. 47)
Hypertonic hand flexor–elbow flexor–shoulder protractor muscle chain	Finger flexor flexibility (p. 81)
Asymmetrical spine and shoulder tension resulting from an asymmetrical posture	Sitting without side bending or twisting (p. 21)
Thoracic spine kyphosis resulting from a posture with cervical spine protraction	Chin tuck mobility (p. 70)
Ergonomic factors that prevent a neutral dynamic spine and shoulder posture	Posture-friendly environment (p. 27)
Hypertonic shoulder elevator and protractor muscles	Relaxed shoulders (p. 45)
Tense pectoral muscles resulting from tension in the jaw muscles	Relaxed lower jaw (p. 41)
Tension in the pectoral muscles caused by a habit of pushing the tongue so far to the front or the side that it touches the teeth	Relaxed tongue (p. 39)
Tension in the pectoral muscles that is associated with a habitually elevated lower lip	Relaxed lower lip (p. 43)
Static holding pattern in the shoulder muscles	Arm swing (p. 62)
Restricted eye movement that is compensated for by an asymmetrical head and shoulder posture	Eye muscle coordination (p. 65)
Holding pattern in the shoulder that can be resolved by cyclical, alternating, and symmetrical movements	Endurance (p. 123)
Forward head posture to compensate for a lack of hip flexion when leaning forward	Stabilized neutral spinal curvature (p. 23)
Blockade of thoracic kinetic chain mobility with shoulder movements due to a habit of keeping the upper body tilted forward or backward	Balanced upper body when seated (p. 25)
Blockade of thoracic kinetic chain mobility with shoulder movements due to a habit of keeping the pelvis shifted forward or backward	Standing posture with a balanced upper body (p. 36)
Habitually static posture	Dynamic sitting and standing (p. 53)

Navigator 12—Sternum and Thorax (chest muscles are excluded)

Potential functional causes of symptoms or dysfunctions	Tests and exercises
Overloading of the thoracic spine and costochondral joints resulting from a slouched sitting posture	Neutral spinal curvature (p. 12)
Thoracic extension deficit	Thoracic extension mobility (p. 73)
Hypomobility of the thoracic spine, ribs, and/or intercostal muscles	Rotational mobility (p. 90)
Thoracic hypomobility resulting from a lack of abdominal breathing or paradoxical breathing	Abdominal breathing (p. 47)
Asymmetrical stress on the spine resulting from an asymmetrical spinal posture	Sitting without side bending or twisting (p. 21)
Overloading of the thoracic spine and sternocostal joints caused by a flexed thoracic spine resulting from weak scapular retractor muscles	Shoulder blade and triceps muscle strength (p. 120)
Ergonomic factors that prevent a neutral dynamic posture with alternation between tension and relaxation	Posture-friendly environment (p. 27)
Habitual shoulder protrusion with synergistic thoracic flexion to compensate for a lack of internal rotation of the glenohumeral joint	Shoulder mobility (p. 78)
Thoracic holding pattern of inspiration	Relaxed shoulders (p. 45)
Thoracic symptoms resulting from holding patterns and/or lack of movement	Endurance (p. 123)
Lack of vertebral stabilization or twisted vertebrae resulting from insufficient or asymmetrical back muscle strength	Back muscle strength (p. 118)
Thoracolumbar flexion and an anterior head posture to compensate for a lack of hip flexion when leaning forward	Stabilized neutral spinal curvature (p. 23)
Muscle imbalance and a nonneutral thoracic spinal posture resulting from an anterior pelvic shift	Standing posture with a balanced upper body (p. 36)
Lack of spinal rotation in walking	Arm swing (p. 62)
Lacking alternation among various seated positions	Changing seated position (p. 50)
Failure to change position	Change of position (p. 51)
Habitually static posture	Dynamic sitting and standing (p. 53)
Thoracic hyperflexion that is promoted by cervical spine protraction	Chin tuck mobility (p. 70)
Muscle imbalance with disproportionate tension in the anterior muscle chain due to a seated position with the upper body leaning backward	Balanced upper body when seated (p. 25)

Navigator 13—Abdomen

Potential functional causes of symptoms or dysfunctions	Tests and exercises
Insufficient mobilization of the abdominal organs resulting from a lack of diaphragmatic movement	Abdominal breathing (p. 47)
Compression of the abdominal organs caused by slouching	Neutral spinal curvature (p. 12)
Compression of the abdominal organs resulting from a thoracic extension deficit	Thoracic extension mobility (p. 73)
Hypomobility of the diaphragm and abdominal organs	Rotational mobility (p. 90)
Slouched sitting posture resulting from insufficient distance between the knees and between the feet	Distance between the knees and between the feet while seated (p. 29)
Abdominal tension that can be resolved by relaxing the tongue	Relaxed tongue (p. 39)
Abdominal tension resulting from a tense lower jaw	Relaxed lower jaw (p. 41)
Abdominal tension resulting from a habit of keeping the lower lip raised	Relaxed lower lip (p. 43)
Abdominal tension that can be resolved by relaxing the shoulders	Relaxed shoulders (p. 45)
Abdominal tension caused by a muscular blockade of spinal rotation while walking	Hip extension (p. 63)
Abdominal symptoms resulting from dysfunction or irritation of the intestines	Endurance (p. 123)
Hypertonicity of the abdominal muscles and/or the iliopsoas	Back muscle strength (p. 118)
Tension or ptosis of the abdominal organs resulting from insufficient or asymmetrical abdominal muscle strength	Abdominal and anterior neck muscle strength (p. 117)
Compression of the abdominal contents resulting from thoracolumbar flexion when leaning forward with insufficient hip flexion	Stabilized neutral spinal curvature (p. 23)
Imbalance between the abdominal and the back muscles	Balanced upper body when seated (p. 25)
Ergonomic factors that prevent a neutral dynamic posture with alternation between tension and relaxation	Posture-friendly environment (p. 27)
Trunk muscle imbalance due to an asymmetrical weight distribution while sitting	Symmetrical weight distribution when sitting (p. 30)
Increased abdominal pressure caused by a flexed thoracic spine, tense abdominal muscles, and pelvic floor resulting from an anterior pelvic shift	Standing posture with a balanced upper body (p. 36)
Static posture habits	Dynamic sitting and standing (p. 53)
Failure to change position	Change of position (p. 51)
Failure to alternate among various seated positions	Changing seated position (p. 50)
Asymmetrical stress of the abdominal muscles and viscera caused by an asymmetrical spinal posture	Sitting without side bending or twisting (p. 21)
Lack of alternate abdominal winding and unwinding resulting from a lack of spinal rotation in walking	Arm swing (p. 62)
Asymmetrical tension in the pelvic floor and iliopsoas muscles resulting from asymmetrical foot placement	Seated posture with symmetrical foot placement (p. 10)

Navigator 14—Lumbar Spine and Buttocks

Potential functional causes of symptoms or dysfunctions	Tests and exercises
Slouched sitting posture	Neutral spinal curvature (p. 12)
Imbalance, consisting of insufficient hip flexion in combination with a lack of lumbar lordosis when leaning forward	Stabilized neutral spinal curvature (p. 23)
Ergonomic factors that prevent a neutral dynamic posture with alternation between tension and relaxation	Posture-friendly environment (p. 27)
Slouched sitting posture resulting from insufficient distance between the knees and between the feet	Distance between the knees and between the feet while seated (p. 29)
Hyperextension of the lumbar spine resulting from a thoracic spine extension deficit Hypertonic abdominal muscles	Thoracic extension mobility (p. 73)
Lumbar hyperextension, compression, and anterior shearing with an extended hip (when standing, walking, and in a supine/prone position with an extended hip) resulting from a hip extension deficit	Hip extension mobility (p. 109)
Flexed lumbar spine in sitting and lifting resulting from shortened hamstring muscles Restricted mobility of the sciatic nerve	Posterior thigh flexibility (p. 101)
Failure to change position	Change of position (p. 51)
Failure to alternate among various sitting positions	Changing seated position (p. 50)
Habitually static posture	Dynamic sitting and standing (p. 53)
Contracted and/or hypertonic diaphragm resulting from chest breathing	Abdominal breathing (p. 47)
Impingement of the sciatic nerve resulting from a contracted or hypertonic piriformis muscle Flexed lumbar spine while sitting to compensate for shortened hip extensors	Buttock muscle flexibility (p. 96)
Uni- or bilateral hip extension deficit resulting from a contracted or hypertonic rectus femoris	Anterior thigh flexibility (p. 113)
Lifting with flexed lumbar spine	Lifting technique (p. 93)
Lumbar instability and hyperextension resulting from insufficient or asymmetrical abdominal muscle strength	Abdominal and anterior neck muscle strength (p. 117)
Lack of vertebral stabilization or twisted vertebrae resulting from insufficient or asymmetrical back muscle strength	Back muscle strength (p. 118)
Restricted neurodynamics of the dura or lumbosacral plexus	Leg, back, and cranial nerve mobility (p. 98)
Restricted rotational mobility of the spine or a lack of internal rotation of the hip	Rotational mobility (p. 90)
Kyphotic lumbar spine while sitting resulting from a seat that is too low	Chair height (p. 28)
Asymmetrical spinal loading due to an asymmetrical weight distribution while sitting	Symmetrical weight distribution when sitting (p. 30)
Imbalance of the spinal muscles because the upper body is leaning too far forward or backward	Balanced upper body when seated (p. 25)
Imbalance of the spinal muscles because the pelvis is shifted too far forward or backward	Standing posture with a balanced upper body (p. 36)

continued on the next page

Navigator 14—Lumbar Spine and Buttocks *(continued)*

Potential functional causes of symptoms or dysfunctions	Tests and exercises
Asymmetrical loading of the spine resulting from an asymmetrical spinal posture	Sitting without side bending or twisting (p. 21)
Sitting up without first rolling to the side	Sitting up (p.58)
Blockade of the kinetic chain in walking resulting from insufficient hip extension	Hip extension (p. 63)
Lack of spinal rotation in walking	Arm swing (p. 62)
Flexed lumbar spine to compensate for a lack of hip flexion	Hip flexion mobility (p. 95)
Asymmetrical stress on the sacroiliac joint and lumbar spine resulting from an asymmetrical foot placement	Seated posture with symmetrical foot placement (p. 10)
Hypertonic posterior muscle chain: leg–hip–lumbar spine Externally rotated hip in walking and standing, caused by insufficient calf flexibility	Calf flexibility (p. 103)
Ipsilateral weight shift and shear load on the pubic symphysis and sacroiliac joint resulting from hypertonic hip adductors	Inner thigh flexibility (p. 106)
Lack of coordination, atrophy, and/or hypertonicity of the hip and trunk muscles resulting from a lack of fine motor control	Balance (p. 60)
Lumbar flexion hypomobility resulting from inflexibility of the back muscles or fascia	Back muscle flexibility (p. 76)
Asymmetrical stress on the sacroiliac joint and lumbar spine resulting from an asymmetrical weight distribution when standing	Symmetrical weight distribution when standing (p. 33)
Hypertonic lumbar spine, hip, and pelvic floor muscles resulting from the base of support being too narrow	Stance width (p. 32)

Navigator 15—Sacroiliac Joint

Potential functional causes of symptoms or dysfunctions	Tests and exercises
Anterior pull of a tense rectus femoris on the ilium, especially if this pull is not equally strong on both sides	Anterior thigh flexibility (p. 113)
Sacroiliac joint compression and anterior torsion of the ilium by a tense iliopsoas, especially if this tension is not equally strong on both sides	Hip extension mobility (p. 109)
Asymmetrical stress on the sacroiliac joint resulting from an asymmetrical foot placement when seated	Seated posture with symmetrical foot placement (p. 10)
Lack of muscular stabilization of the iliosacral joint resulting from a slouched sitting posture	Neutral spinal curvature (p. 12)
Sacroiliac torsion caused by crossing the legs Sacroiliac stress from a hypertonic iliopsoas due to sitting with the knees too close together	Distance between the knees and between the feet while seated (p. 29)
Asymmetrical sacroiliac loading due to an asymmetrical weight distribution when sitting	Symmetrical weight distribution when sitting (p. 30)
Hyperextension of the lumbar spine resulting from a thoracic extension deficit Hypertonic abdominal muscles	Thoracic extension mobility (p. 73)
Pull of tight hamstring muscles on the ischial tuberosity, especially when the pull is not equally strong on both sides Sacroiliac joint hypermobility to compensate for a lack of hip flexion	Posterior thigh flexibility (p. 101)
Malpositioning of the sacrum resulting from a tense piriformis muscle Sacroiliac hypermobility as compensation for a lack of internal hip rotation	Buttock muscle flexibility (p. 96)
Sacroiliac hypermobility resulting from a lack of muscular stabilization when leaning forward or backward	Stabilized neutral spinal curvature (p. 23)
Asymmetrical stress on the sacroiliac joint due to an asymmetrical weight distribution when standing	Symmetrical weight distribution when standing (p. 33)
Stress on the sacroiliac joint resulting from a static posture	Dynamic sitting and standing (p. 53)
Muscular imbalance and a nonneutral sacroiliac joint position resulting from an anterior pelvic shift	Standing posture with a balanced upper body (p. 36)
Lumbosacral instability and hyperextension resulting from insufficient or asymmetrical abdominal muscle strength	Abdominal and anterior neck muscle strength (p. 117)
Excessive stress on the sacroiliac joint resulting from sitting up without first rolling to the side	Sitting up (p. 58)
Blockade of the sacroiliac joint and/or a tight piriformis muscle	Rotational mobility (p. 90)
Sacroiliac instability or twisting resulting from insufficient or asymmetrical back muscle strength	Back muscle strength (p. 118)
Blockade of the kinetic chain in walking resulting from a lack of hip extension	Hip extension (p. 63)
Ergonomic factors that prevent a neutral dynamic posture with alternation between tension and relaxation	Posture-friendly environment (p. 27)
Failure to change position	Change of position (p. 51)
Asymmetrical stress on the sacroiliac joint resulting from an asymmetrical spinal posture	Sitting without side bending or twisting (p. 21)

continued on the next page

Navigator 15—Sacroiliac Joint *(continued)*

Potential functional causes of symptoms or dysfunctions	Tests and exercises
Failure to alternate among various sitting positions	Changing seated position (p. 50)
Lack of spinal rotation in walking	Arm swing (p. 62)
Flexed lumbar spine due to sitting on a seat that is too low	Chair height (p. 28)
Ipsilateral weight shift and shear load on the pubic symphysis and sacroiliac joint resulting from insufficient flexibility of the hip adductors	Inner thigh flexibility (p. 106)
Imbalance of the trunk muscles when the upper body leans too far forward or backward when seated	Balanced upper body when seated (p. 25)
Iliosacral tightness that can be resolved by repeated, cyclical, alternating, and symmetrical movements	Endurance (p. 123)
Hypertonic lumbar spine, hip, and pelvic floor muscles when the base of support is too narrow	Stance width (p. 32)
Tension in the pelvic floor and trunk that can be resolved by abdominal breathing	Abdominal breathing (p. 47)
Sacroiliac joint hypermobility resulting from hip flexion hypomobility	Hip flexion mobility (p. 95)
Excessive sacroiliac stress due to a lifting technique with too much lumbosacral flexion	Lifting technique (p. 93)
Tight sacroiliac muscles due to restricted neurodynamics in the dura or lumbosacral plexus	Leg, back, and cranial nerve mobility (p. 98)
Hypertonic posterior muscle chain: leg–hip–lumbar spine	Calf flexibility (p. 103)
Externally rotated hip position in walking and standing caused by insufficient calf flexibility	
Lack of lumbosacral flexion mobility resulting from deficient flexibility of the back muscles or fascia	Back muscle flexibility (p. 76)
Deficient coordination or hypertonicity of the hip and trunk muscles	Balance (p. 60)
Sacroiliac tightness that can be resolved by relaxed shoulders	Relaxed shoulders (p. 45)
Sacroiliac tightness that can be resolved by lower jaw relaxation	Relaxed lower jaw (p. 41)
Sacroiliac tightness that can be resolved by tongue relaxation	Relaxed tongue (p. 39)
Sacroiliac tightness resulting from a habit of keeping the lower lip raised	Relaxed lower lip (p. 43)

Navigator 16—Lateral Thigh

Potential functional causes of symptoms or dysfunctions	Tests and exercises
Compression of the lateral femoral cutaneous nerve in the muscular lacuna and tightness of the tensor fasciae latae as a result of an anterior pelvic shift	Standing posture with a balanced upper body (p. 36)
Insufficient flexibility of the tensor fasciae latae and iliopsoas Compression of the lateral femoral cutaneous nerve in the muscular lacuna	Hip extension mobility (p. 109)
Tightness of the iliopsoas to balance the torque of a backward-leaning upper body when seated	Balanced upper body when seated (p. 25)
Tightness of the iliopsoas muscle resulting from a habit of keeping the heels raised while sitting	Symmetrical weight distribution when sitting (p. 30)
Overloaded hip joint and fascia lata in the habitually weight-bearing leg	Symmetrical weight distribution when standing (p. 33)
Insufficient flexibility of the anterior thigh and anterior portions of the fascia lata	Anterior thigh flexibility (p. 113)
Tension in the hip flexor, pelvic floor, or abdominal muscles that can be resolved by abdominal breathing	Abdominal breathing (p. 47)
Nerve compression caused by a poor lifting technique, either peripherally in the muscular lacuna or centrally by the lumbar disks	Lifting technique (p. 93)
Ergonomic factors that prevent a neutral dynamic posture with alternation between tension and relaxation	Posture-friendly environment (p. 27)
Flexed lumbar spine, compression in the groin, and hypertonic iliopsoas caused by a seat that is too low	Chair height (p. 28)
Twisted sacroiliac joint and tension in the iliopsoas caused by sitting with crossed legs	Distance between the knees and between the feet while seated (p. 29)
Overloading of the lumbar spine and the hip joint caused by a static posture while sitting	Changing seated position (p. 50)
Overloading of the lumbar spine and the hip joint caused by a failure to change position	Change of position (p. 51)
Overloading of the lumbar spine and hip joint caused by a static standing and sitting posture	Dynamic sitting and standing (p. 53)
Blockade of the kinetic chain in walking resulting from a lack of hip extension	Hip extension (p. 63)
Stress on the sacroiliac joint and lumbar spine caused by sitting up without first rolling to the side	Sitting up (p. 58)
Overloading of the fascia lata and hip joint resulting from tight buttock muscles	Buttock muscle flexibility (p. 96)
Hip joint dysfunction resulting from insufficient flexibility of the hip adductors	Inner thigh flexibility (p. 106)

Navigator 17—Anterior Thigh

Potential functional causes of symptoms or dysfunctions	Tests and exercises
Lack of flexibility in the anterior thigh	Anterior thigh flexibility (p. 113)
Irritation in the groin and hip joint resulting from an anterior pelvic shift	Standing posture with a balanced upper body (p. 36)
Tight knee extensors as a cause or result of an asymmetrical weight distribution while sitting	Symmetrical weight distribution when sitting (p. 30)
Increased tension in the rectus femoris and sartorius muscles to balance the torque of a backward-leaning upper body	Balanced upper body when seated (p. 25)
Lack of flexibility in the hip flexors	Hip extension mobility (p. 109)
Blockade of the kinetic chain in walking resulting from a lack of hip extension	Hip extension (p. 63)
Increased tension in the rectus femoris and sartorius muscles to hold the pelvis upright in spite of an adducted leg position when seated	Distance between the knees and between the feet while seated (p. 29)
Increased tension in the rectus femoris and sartorius muscles to hold the pelvis upright in spite of a seat that is too low	Chair height (p. 28)
Hypertonicity of the rectus femoris and sartorius muscles resulting from sacroiliac joint dysfunction	Rotational mobility (p. 90)
Ergonomic factors that prevent a neutral dynamic posture with alternation between tension and relaxation	Posture-friendly environment (p. 27)
Dysfunction of the quadriceps in walking and standing resulting from a limited calf flexibility that restricts dorsiflexion of the talocrural joint	Calf flexibility (p. 103)
Increased tension in the rectus femoris and sartorius muscles resulting from a sacroiliac joint dysfunction or in order to hold the pelvis upright while sitting, in spite of deficient buttock flexibility	Buttock muscle flexibility (p. 96)
Increased tension in the rectus femoris and sartorius muscles resulting from a sacroiliac joint dysfunction or in order to compensate for deficient hamstring flexibility	Posterior thigh flexibility (p. 101)
Overuse of the quadriceps femoris on the habitually weight-bearing side	Symmetrical weight distribution when standing (p. 33)
Overuse of the knee, hip, and thigh muscles by insufficient changing of position	Change of position (p. 51)
Increased tension in the thigh resulting from a sacroiliac joint dysfunction or from sitting with the feet placed or hooked under the chair	Seated posture with symmetrical foot placement (p. 10)
Sacroiliac joint dysfunction resulting from insufficient flexibility of the hip adductors	Inner thigh flexibility (p. 106)
Tightness of the hip flexor, pelvic floor, or abdominal muscles that can be resolved by abdominal breathing	Abdominal breathing (p. 47)
Overuse of the knee joint, hip joint, and thigh muscles resulting from a static posture in standing or sitting	Dynamic sitting and standing (p. 53)
Asymmetrical use of the knee joint, hip joint, and thigh muscles resulting from a lack of variation in seated posture	Changing seated position (p. 50)

Navigator 18—Medial Thigh

Potential functional causes of symptoms or dysfunctions	Tests and exercises
Insufficient hip adductor flexibility	Inner thigh flexibility (p. 106)
Sitting with the knees too close together	Distance between the knees and between the feet while seated (p. 29)
Hypertonic or shortened hip adductors due to iliopsoas tightness	Hip extension mobility (p. 109)
Tense hip adductors resulting from dysfunction in the sacroiliac joint	Anterior thigh flexibility (p. 113)
Tense hip adductors resulting from an asymmetrical weight distribution while sitting	Symmetrical weight distribution when sitting (p. 30)
Sacroiliac dysfunction resulting from standing with the weight always on the same leg	Symmetrical weight distribution when standing (p. 33)
Tense hip adductors resulting from sacroiliac dysfunction or a posture with asymmetrical hip abduction or adduction	Seated posture with symmetrical foot placement (p. 10)
Blockade of the kinetic chain in walking resulting from tension in the hip flexors and adductors	Hip extension (p. 63)
Walking with excessive external rotation of the hip caused by insufficient calf flexibility	Calf flexibility (p. 103)
Irritation of the obturator nerve resulting from excessive lumbar flexion to compensate for insufficient hamstring flexibility	Posterior thigh flexibility (p. 101)
Irritation of the obturator nerve as a result of excessive lumbar spine flexion to compensate for insufficient buttock muscle flexibility	Buttock muscle flexibility (p. 96)

Navigator 19—Dorsal Thigh

Potential functional causes of symptoms or dysfunctions	Tests and exercises
Restricted neurodynamics of the sciatic nerve or insufficient flexibility of the hamstring muscles	Posterior thigh flexibility (p. 101)
Restricted neurodynamics of the dura or sciatic nerve	Leg, back, and cranial nerve mobility (p. 98)
Dysfunction of the muscles and nerves of the posterior thigh resulting from an insufficient stabilization of lumbar spine lordosis	Stabilized neutral spinal curvature (p. 23)
Poor lifting technique resulting in dysfunction of the lumbar disks or the sacroiliac joint and subsequent muscle or nerve irritation in the posterior thigh	Lifting technique (p. 93)
Lumbar spine instability or insufficient flexibility of the posterior thigh resulting from sitting with a flexed lumbar spine	Neutral spinal curvature (p. 12)
Lumbar spine instability or insufficient flexibility of the hamstring muscles resulting from insufficient hip flexion	Hip flexion mobility (p. 95)
Lumbar spine instability or entrapment of the sciatic nerve under the piriformis muscle resulting from insufficient buttock muscle flexibility	Buttock muscle flexibility (p. 96)
Hypertonic posterior muscle chain: leg–hip–lumbar spine	Calf flexibility (p. 103).
Blockade of the kinetic chain in walking resulting from a hip extension deficit	Hip extension (p. 63)
Dysfunction of the lumbar spine, sacroiliac joint, hip, or knee resulting from a hip extension deficit	Hip extension mobility (p. 109)
Dysfunction of the lumbar spine, sacroiliac joint, or hip resulting from insufficient flexibility of the anterior thigh	Anterior thigh flexibility (p. 113)
Irritation of the nerve roots of the sciatic nerve in the area of the lumbar disks resulting from sitting up without first rolling to the side	Sitting up (p. 58)
Overloading of the lumbar spine, hip, and knee caused by a failure to change position	Change of position (p. 51)
Overloading of the lumbar spine, hip, and knee caused by a lack of changing seated position	Changing seated position (p. 50)
Overloading of the lumbar spine, hip, and knee, caused by a static standing or sitting position	Dynamic sitting and standing (p. 53)
Asymmetrical stress on the sacroiliac joint and hamstring muscles resulting from an asymmetrical knee or hip joint angle	Seated posture with symmetrical foot placement (p. 10)

Navigator 20—Knee

Potential functional causes of symptoms or dysfunctions	Tests and exercises
Increased patellofemoral contact pressure or malalignment resulting from insufficient flexibility of the anterior thigh	Anterior thigh flexibility (p. 113)
Increased patellofemoral contact pressure or malalignment resulting from insufficient flexibility of the posterior thigh	Posterior thigh flexibility (p. 101)
Lateralization of the patella resulting from insufficient flexibility of the fascia lata and iliotibial band or walking with too much external hip rotation	Rotational mobility (p. 90)
Dysfunction of the tibiofemoral or patellofemoral joint resulting from walking with too much external hip rotation due to insufficient calf flexibility	Calf flexibility (p. 103)
Increased patellofemoral contact pressure resulting from a seat that is too low	Chair height (p. 28)
Cartilage dysfunction of the knees resulting from insufficient change of position	Change of position (p. 51)
Blockade of physiological knee movements at the end of the stance phase due to insufficient hip extension mobility	Hip extension mobility (p. 109)
Gait with excessive external hip rotation resulting from insufficient buttock muscle flexibility	Buttock muscle flexibility (p. 96)
Insufficient knee control when, for example, the knee takes on a valgus position in the stance phase	Balance (p. 60)
Insufficient knee control in lifting when the base of support and balance are decreased as a result of lifting the heel	Lifting technique (p. 93)
Blockade of physiological knee movements at the end of the stance phase as a result of insufficient hip extension	Hip extension (p. 63)
Lateralization of the patella resulting from sitting with an insufficient distance between the knees	Distance between the knees and between the feet while seated (p. 29)
Hyperextension of the knees resulting from an anterior pelvic shift	Standing posture with a balanced upper body (p. 36)
Varus stress on the knees resulting from sitting with crossed legs	Seated posture with symmetrical foot placement (p. 10)
Insufficient nourishment of the cartilage, menisci, and muscles resulting from a static standing and sitting posture	Dynamic sitting and standing (p. 53)
Increased patellofemoral contact pressure resulting from tightness of the rectus femoris muscle when trying to support an upper body that is tilted too far backward	Balanced upper body when seated (p. 25)
Overloading the knee on the habitually weight-bearing leg	Symmetrical weight distribution when standing (p. 33)
Valgus stress of the knees and tibial internal rotation resulting from a stance that is too wide	Stance width (p. 32)
Excessive external rotation of the femur on the tibia at the end of the stance phase due to an insufficient counterswing of the ipsilateral arm	Arm swing (p. 62)
Ergonomic factors that prevent a neutral dynamic posture of the knee	Posture-friendly environment (p. 27)
Insufficient posterior thigh flexibility due to a lack of hip flexion when leaning forward	Stabilized neutral spinal curvature (p. 23)
Tense hip extensors and knee flexors resulting from restricted neurodynamics of the sciatic nerve	Leg, back, and cranial nerve mobility (p. 98)
Short hamstrings resulting from sitting with a flexed lumbar spine	Neutral spinal curvature (p. 12)
Asymmetrical stress on the knees due to an asymmetrical weight distribution while sitting	Symmetrical weight distribution when sitting (p. 30)

Navigator 21—Lateral Aspect of the Lower Leg

Potential functional causes of symptoms or dysfunctions	Tests and exercises
Lack of toe and foot elevator flexibility (tibialis anterior, extensor digitorum, extensor hallucis longus, and peroneus tertius)	Anterior thigh flexibility (p. 113)
Overuse of the dorsiflexors by habitually bearing more weight on the ipsilateral side or shifting the weight too far toward the heel	Symmetrical weight distribution when standing (p. 33)
Excessive pronation of the subtalar joint in the stance phase or when squatting to compensate for lack of calf flexibility	Calf flexibility (p. 103)
Tense toe and foot elevators resulting from or causing an asymmetrical weight distribution when sitting, e. g., when a foot pedal is operated	Symmetrical weight distribution when sitting (p. 30)
Talocrural dorsiflexion hypomobility that must be compensated for by excessive tension in the dorsiflexors while squatting	Lifting technique (p. 93)
A lack of tibial external rotation at the end of the stance phase resulting from insufficient hip extension	Hip extension (p. 63)
A lack of tibial external rotation at the end of the stance phase resulting from hip extension hypomobility	Hip extension mobility (p. 109)
Increased tension in the dorsiflexors to balance the torque of a backward-leaning upper body	Balanced upper body when seated (p. 25)
Tense dorsiflexors to compensate for a lack of physiological rotation in walking	Arm swing (p. 62)
Tense tibialis anterior resulting from excessive subtalar pronation in the stance phase due to deficient balance	Balance (p. 60)
Synergistic tension in the dorsiflexors when the hip flexors have to compensate for the hip extension torque that is generated by a seat which is too low	Chair height (p. 28)
Synergistic tension in the dorsiflexors when the hip flexor muscles must contract to compensate for the hip extension torque that is generated by a posture with crossed legs	Seated posture with symmetrical foot placement (p. 10)
Tension in the tibialis anterior to prevent increased pronation in the subtalar joint when walking with an externally rotated hip	Buttock muscle flexibility (p. 96)
Insufficient circulation in the dorsiflexors resulting from static tension	Dynamic sitting and standing (p. 53)
Tense tibialis anterior to prevent the increased pronation that results from an excessively wide stance	Stance width (p. 32)

Navigator 22—Calf

Potential functional causes of symptoms or dysfunctions	Tests and exercises
Tight calf muscles	Calf flexibility (p. 103)
Tension and pain in the calves resulting from restricted neurodynamics of the sciatic nerve	Leg, back, and cranial nerve mobility (p. 98)
Decreased neurodynamics of the sciatic nerve resulting from lumbar disk dysfunction or adhesion of the sciatic nerve to the hamstring muscles	Posterior thigh flexibility (p. 101)
Overloading of the calf muscles and veins caused by a static standing and sitting posture	Dynamic sitting and standing (p. 53)
Blockade of physiological gait in the stance phase resulting from insufficient hip extension	Hip extension (p. 63)
Gait with excessive external hip rotation resulting from insufficient buttock muscle flexibility	Buttock muscle flexibility (p. 96)
Tension and pain in the calf muscles caused by irritation of the sciatic nerve in the region of the lumbar disks due to a poor lifting technique	Lifting technique (p. 93)
Blockade of physiological gait in the stance phase as a result of insufficient hip extension	Hip extension mobility (p. 109)
Asymmetrical calf muscle tension resulting from an asymmetrical weight distribution while sitting	Symmetrical weight distribution when sitting (p. 30)
Unphysiological gait in the stance phase resulting from an insufficient arm swing	Arm swing (p. 62)
Overuse of the calf muscles on the habitually weight-bearing leg	Symmetrical weight distribution when standing (p. 33)
Pronation of the subtalar joint resulting from an excessively wide stance	Stance width (p. 32)
Unilateral stress on the calf muscles and veins resulting from a failure to change position	Change of position (p. 51)
Irritation of the sciatic nerve in the area of the lumbar spine, piriformis, or hamstrings resulting from slouched sitting	Neutral spinal curvature (p. 12)
Irritation of the sciatic nerve in the area of the lumbar spine, piriformis, or hamstrings resulting from a lack of lumbar spine stabilization when leaning forward	Stabilized neutral spinal curvature (p. 23)
Calf muscles tightness resulting from a habit of shifting the body's center of gravity too far forward	Standing posture with a balanced upper body (p. 36)
Obstruction of the venous return from the calf by a seat that is too high or too low	Chair height (p. 28)

Navigator 23—Feet

Potential functional causes of symptoms or dysfunctions	Tests and exercises
Stress on the arch of the foot resulting from insufficient calf flexibility	Calf flexibility (p. 103)
Static stress on the arch resulting from lack of position change	Change of position (p. 51)
Irritation of the nerve roots of L4–S2 in the lumbar disk region resulting from a poor lifting technique	Lifting technique (p. 93)
Stress on the arch caused by a static standing and sitting posture	Dynamic sitting and standing (p. 53)
Excessive stress on the foot muscles and joints of the habitually weight-bearing leg	Symmetrical weight distribution when standing (p. 33)
Pronation of the feet resulting from an excessively wide stance	Stance width (p. 32)
Overloading of the arches and foot muscles resulting from an insufficient balance reaction in the stance phase	Balance (p. 60)
Increased external rotation of the hip when walking, with overloading of the transverse arch of the foot because of a lack of buttock muscle flexibility	Buttock muscle flexibility (p. 96)
Blockade of physiological gait in the stance phase caused by insufficient hip extension	Hip extension (p. 63)
Blockade of physiological gait in the stance phase as a result of insufficient hip extension mobility	Hip extension mobility (p. 109)
Lack of dorsiflexor flexibility (anterior tibial, extensor digitorum, extensor hallucis longus, and peroneus tertius)	Anterior thigh flexibility (p. 113)
Unphysiological gait in the stance phase due to a lack of arm swing	Arm swing (p. 62)
Asymmetrical tension in the foot muscles due to an asymmetrical weight distribution while sitting	Symmetrical weight distribution when sitting (p. 30)
Foot dysfunction due to a nonneutral foot placement	Seated posture with symmetrical foot placement (p. 10)
Foot dysfunction resulting from shifting the body's center of gravity too far backward or forward	Balanced upper body when seated (p. 25)
Pronation stress on the feet resulting from excessive dorsal talocrural extension because of a seat that is too low	Chair height (p. 28)
Ergonomic factors that prevent a neutral dynamic posture of the feet with alternation between loading and unloading	Posture-friendly environment (p. 27)
Tension and pain in the feet resulting from restricted neurodynamics of the sciatic nerve	Leg, back, and cranial nerve mobility (p. 98)

Navigator 24—Cervical Spine—Radiating to the Arm and Hand

Potential functional causes of symptoms or dysfunctions	Tests and exercises
Sitting with forward head posture	Neutral spinal curvature (p. 12)
Cervical spine hyperextension resulting from thoracic spine extension hypomobility	Thoracic extension mobility (p. 73)
Restricted cervical spine retraction mobility	Chin tuck mobility (p. 70)
Hypertonic shoulder and neck muscles resulting from chest breathing	Abdominal breathing (p. 47)
Hypertonic shoulder elevator muscles	Relaxed shoulders (p. 45)
Asymmetrical stress on the spine resulting from an asymmetrical spinal posture	Sitting without side bending or twisting (p. 21)
Forward head position to compensate for insufficient hip flexion when leaning forward	Stabilized neutral spinal curvature (p. 23)
Hypertonic shoulder elevator and protractor muscles resulting from restricted neurodynamics of the brachial plexus	Arm nerve mobility (p. 83)
Shoulder protraction, brachial plexus hypomobility, and/or insufficient thoracic spine extension resulting from tight pectoral muscles	Rotational mobility (p. 90)
Hypertonic muscle chain: hand flexor–elbow flexors–shoulder protractor	Finger flexor flexibility (p. 81)
Ergonomic factors that prevent a neutral dynamic posture with alternation between tension and relaxation	Posture-friendly environment (p. 27)
Restricted eye movement compensated for by asymmetrical cervical tension	Eye muscle coordination (p. 65)
Tension in the neck muscles resulting from tension in the jaw muscles	Relaxed lower jaw (p. 41)
Tension in the neck muscles caused by a habit of pushing the tongue so far to the front or the side that it touches the teeth	Relaxed tongue (p. 39)
Tension in the neck muscles that is associated with a habitually elevated lower lip	Relaxed lower lip (p. 43)
Habitual static posture	Dynamic sitting and standing (p. 53)
Restricted dural neurodynamics	Leg, back, and cranial nerve mobility (p. 98)
Failure to change position	Change of position (p. 51)
Habitual shoulder protrusion to compensate for a lack of internal rotation of the glenohumeral joint	Shoulder mobility (p. 78)
Habitual shoulder protrusion resulting from weak scapular retractor muscles	Shoulder blade and triceps muscle strength (p. 120)
Insufficient vertebral stabilization or twisted vertebrae resulting from insufficient or asymmetrical back muscle strength	Back muscle strength (p. 118)
Imbalance between tense neck extensors and hypotonic cervical spine flexors	Abdominal and anterior neck muscle strength (p. 117)
Muscular imbalance and a nonneutral cervical spine posture resulting from an anterior pelvic shift	Standing posture with a balanced upper body (p. 36)
Imbalance of the trunk muscles because the upper body is leaning too far forward or backward while sitting	Balanced upper body when seated (p. 25)
Lack of spinal rotation in walking	Arm swing (p. 62)

continued on the next page

Navigator 24—Cervical Spine—Radiating to the Arm and Hand *(continued)*

Potential functional causes of symptoms or dysfunctions	Tests and exercises
Excessive spinal S-curve when standing resulting from insufficient hip extension	Hip extension mobility (p. 109)
Slouched sitting position because of a seat that is too low	Chair height (p. 28)
Slouched sitting position because the distance between the knees is too small	Distance between the knees and between the feet while seated (p. 29)
Asymmetrical stress on the cervical spine resulting from an asymmetrical weight distribution while sitting	Symmetrical weight distribution when sitting (p. 30)
Lack of alternation among various seated positions	Changing seated position (p. 50)
Slouched sitting position resulting from restricted hamstring flexibility	Posterior thigh flexibility (p. 101)

Navigator 25—Lumbar Spine—Radiating to the Leg and Foot

Potential functional causes of symptoms or dysfunctions	Tests and exercises
Sitting with a flexed lumbar spine	Neutral spinal curvature (p. 12)
Lifting with a flexed lumbar spine	Lifting technique (p. 93)
Sitting up without first rolling to the side	Sitting up (p. 58)
Flexed lumbar spine in sitting and lifting resulting from a lack of hamstring flexibility	Posterior thigh flexibility (p. 101)
Restricted neurodynamics of the sciatic nerve resulting from adhesion of the sciatic nerve to the hamstring muscles	
Impingement and restricted neurodynamics of the sciatic nerve resulting from a short or hypertonic piriformis muscle	Buttock muscle flexibility (p. 96)
Slouched sitting position due to tight hip extensors	
Restricted neurodynamics of the dura or the lumbosacral plexus	Leg, back, and cranial nerve mobility (p. 98)
Hyperextension, compression, and an anterior shearing load on the lumbar spine with an extended hip (standing, walking, and a supine/prone position with an extended hip) resulting from tight hip flexors	Hip extension mobility (p. 109)
Hypertonic posterior muscle chain: leg–hip–lumbar spine	Calf flexibility (p. 103)
External rotated hip position in walking and standing resulting from a muscular restriction of lack of calf flexibility	
Uni- or bilateral pull of a short or hypertonic rectus femoris on the ilium, especially in postures with hip extension and knee flexion	Anterior thigh flexibility (p. 113)
Hyperextension of the lumbar spine while standing resulting from insufficient thoracic spine extension mobility	Thoracic extension mobility (p. 73)
Weak abdominal muscles	
Failure to change position	Change of position (p. 51)
Lack of alternation among various seated positions	Changing seated position (p. 50)
Habitually static posture	Dynamic sitting and standing (p. 53)
Ergonomic factors that prevent a neutral dynamic posture with alternation between loading and unloading	Posture-friendly environment (p. 27)
Insufficient vertebral stabilization or twisted vertebrae resulting from insufficient or asymmetrical back muscle strength	Back muscle strength (p. 118)
Insufficient vertebral stabilization and lumbar spine hyperextension resulting from insufficient or asymmetrical abdominal muscle strength	Abdominal and anterior neck muscle strength (p. 117)
Insufficient flexibility in the back muscles and fasciae	Back muscle flexibility (p. 76)
Tight diaphragm resulting from chest breathing	Abdominal breathing (p. 47)
Lumbar spine hyperextension resulting from an anterior pelvic shift while standing	Standing posture with a balanced upper body (p. 36)
Hypermobility of the sacroiliac joint and posterior lumbar disks to compensate for a lack of hip flexion when leaning forward	Stabilized neutral spinal curvature (p. 23)
Slouched sitting position resulting from a seat that is too low	Chair height (p. 28)
Slouched sitting position resulting from an insufficient distance between the knees	Distance between the knees and between the feet while seated (p. 29)
Limited rotational mobility	Rotational mobility (p. 90)
Flexed lumbar spine resulting from insufficient hip flexion	Hip flexion mobility (p. 95)

continued on the next page

Navigator 25—Lumbar Spine—Radiating to the Leg and Foot *(continued)*

Potential functional causes of symptoms or dysfunctions	Tests and exercises
Asymmetrical spinal loading resulting from an asymmetrical weight distribution while sitting	Symmetrical weight distribution when sitting (p. 30)
Blockade of the physiological kinetic chain in walking resulting from a hip extension deficit	Hip extension (p. 63)
Asymmetrical stress on the spine resulting from an asymmetrical spinal posture	Sitting without side bending or twisting (p. 21)
Imbalance of the spine-stabilizing muscles because the upper body is leaning too far forward or backward	Balanced upper body when seated (p. 25)
Lack of spinal counterrotation in walking resulting from a lack of arm swing	Arm swing (p. 62)
Restricted neurodynamics of the upper extremity, which also hampers the neurodynamics of the lumbar spine and leg nerves	Arm nerve mobility (p. 83)

Navigator 26—Twisted or Hypomobile Vertebrae

Twisted or hypomobile vertebrae C0–C5

Potential functional causes of symptoms or dysfunctions	Tests and exercises
Tension in the neck muscles caused by a habit of pushing the tongue so far to the front or the side that it touches the teeth	Relaxed tongue (p. 39)
Tension in the neck muscles because of tension in the jaw muscles	Relaxed lower jaw (p. 41)
Hypertonic shoulder elevator muscles	Relaxed shoulders (p. 45)
Hypertonic shoulder and neck muscles resulting from chest breathing	Abdominal breathing (p. 47)
Hypertonic neck extensor muscles and tension in the ligamentous attachment of the dura to the vertebrae as a result of restricted dural neurodynamics	Leg, back, and cranial nerve mobility (p. 98)
Insufficient muscular stabilization of the vertebrae due to a slouched sitting posture	Neutral spinal curvature (p. 12)
Tension in the neck muscles that is associated with a habitually elevated lower lip	Relaxed lower lip (p. 43)
Twisted vertebrae resulting from a twisted posture	Sitting without side bending or twisting (p. 21)
Ergonomic factors that prevent a neutral dynamic posture	Posture-friendly environment (p. 27)

Twisted or hypomobile vertebrae C6–T3 (cervicothoracic junction)

Potential functional causes of symptoms or dysfunctions	Tests and exercises
Scapular protraction resulting from insufficient flexibility of the pectoral muscles	Rotational mobility (p. 90)
Cervical spine hyperextension resulting from insufficient thoracic spine extension	Thoracic extension mobility (p. 73)
Hypertonic ipsilateral cervical spine muscles and pull of hypomobile nerves at their attachment in the intervertebral foramina	Arm nerve mobility (p. 83)
Hypertonic neck extensors and tension in the ligamentous attachment of the dura to the vertebrae as a result of restricted dural neurodynamics	Leg, back, and cranial nerve mobility (p. 98)
Twisted vertebrae resulting from a twisted posture	Sitting without side bending or twisting (p. 21)
Sitting with a forward head posture	Neutral spinal curvature (p. 12)
Ergonomic factors that prevent a neutral dynamic posture with alternation between tension and relaxation	Posture-friendly environment (p. 27)
Hypertonic shoulder and neck muscles resulting from chest breathing	Abdominal breathing (p. 47)
Hypertonic shoulder elevator muscles	Relaxed shoulders (p. 45)
Tension in the neck muscles because of tension in the jaw muscles	Relaxed lower jaw (p. 41)
Tension in the neck muscles caused by a habit of pushing the tongue so far to the front or the side that it touches the teeth	Relaxed tongue (p. 39)
Tension in the neck muscles that is associated with a habitually elevated lower lip	Relaxed lower lip (p. 43)

Twisted or hypomobile vertebrae T6–T10 (where a bra strap would be and immediately above)

Potential functional causes of symptoms or dysfunctions	Tests and exercises
Tension in the diaphragm with chest or paradoxical breathing	Abdominal breathing (p. 47)
Insufficient muscular stabilization of the vertebrae due to a slouched sitting posture	Neutral spinal curvature (p. 12)
Twisted vertebrae as a result of a twisted posture	Sitting without side bending or twisting (p. 21)

Twisted or hypomobile vertebrae in the lumbar spine

Potential functional causes of symptoms or dysfunctions	Tests and exercises
Insufficient muscular stabilization of the vertebrae due to a slouched sitting posture	Neutral spinal curvature (p. 12)
Twisted vertebrae as a result of a twisted posture	Sitting without side bending or twisting (p. 21)
Ergonomic factors that prevent a neutral dynamic posture	Posture-friendly environment (p. 27)
Insufficient muscular stabilization of the vertebrae when leaning	Stabilized neutral spinal curvature (p. 23)
Twisted vertebrae as a result of a malaligned sacroiliac joint	Anterior thigh flexibility (p. 113)
Twisted vertebrae as a result of sacroiliac dysfunction or direct traction of a tight psoas muscle on vertebrae L1–L5	Hip extension mobility (p. 109)

13 Measuring + Planning + Communicating

13.1 How To Measure Progress toward the Test Goal

▶ **Posture, relaxation, movement, and coordination.** A subjective estimate of the percentage of the day (with the exception of sleep time) during which the patient achieves the goal during everyday activities.

▶ **Abdominal and back muscle strength.** The number of repetitions that can be performed slowly, smoothly, and without trembling, pain, or considerable exertion.

▶ **Shoulder blade and triceps muscle strength.** The number of seconds for which the position can be held steadily, without trembling, pain, or considerable exertion.

▶ **Endurance.** The average number of minutes of endurance training per week that can be accomplished with a pulse rate of about 120 beats per minute while experiencing a subjective feeling of well-being.

▶ **Mobility.** The distance from the test goal in finger widths (**Figs. 13.1**, **13.2**, **13.3**) or centimeters (**Figs. 13.4–13.12**).

13.1.1 Measurement in Finger Widths

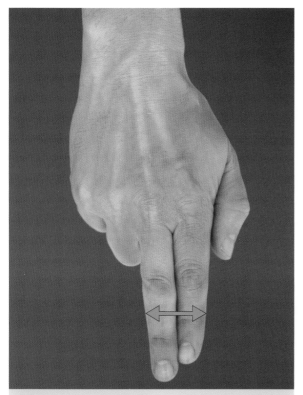

Fig. 13.1 Two fingers wide.

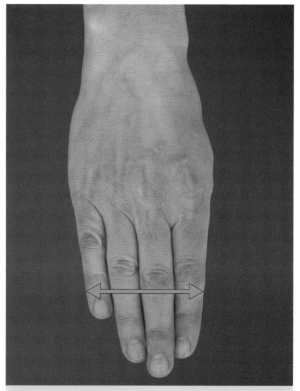

Fig. 13.2 Four fingers wide.

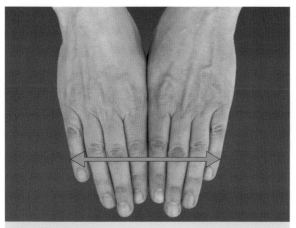

Fig. 13.3 Eight fingers wide.

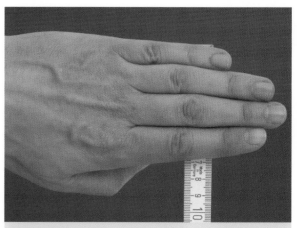

Fig. 13.4 Measurement of finger widths with a ruler.

13.1.2 Measurement in Centimeters

There are two possibilities for measurement in centimeters.

▶ **Measuring the fingers.** After measuring the distance from the test goal in finger widths, the therapist reads off the width of the fingers on a ruler (**Fig. 13.4**) or a caliper gauge (**Fig. 13.5**) in centimeters.

▶ **Measuring with a folding ruler.** Small distances can be measured with a common folding ruler that consists of a number of hinged sections. The distance to the test goal can be measured in five specific widths as follows: a typical metric 2-m folding ruler is composed of 10 sections, each 3.5 mm thick, resulting in a total width of 3.5 cm. It is easiest to measure with the end of the folding ruler at which all 10 sections are equally long (**Fig. 13.6**). At this end, there are always two sections riveted to each other, so that, with a ruler that is 3.5 cm wide, the five double sections each have a width of 7 mm. To avoid having to undertake mental arithmetic, the five 7-mm widths can be marked on the ruler (**Fig. 13.7**).

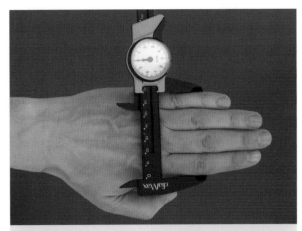

Fig. 13.5 Measurement of finger widths with a caliper gauge.

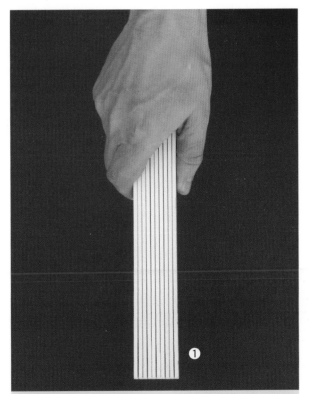

Fig. 13.6 A common folding ruler in which all 10 sections are equally long on one side, ①.

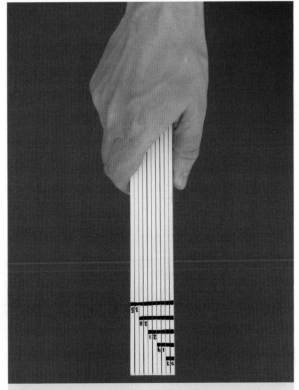

Fig. 13.7 A folding ruler on which five different widths have been marked.

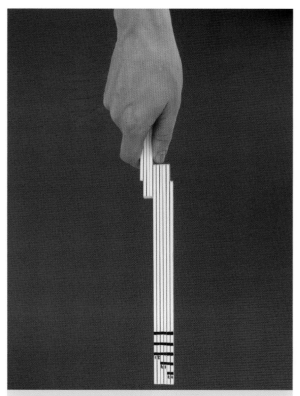

Fig. 13.8 An unfolded 21-mm wide block ...

For the measurement, the patient moves toward the test goal until she feels the onset of tension and remains in this position. If at this point she has not yet reached the test goal, the therapist estimates the distance from the test goal, unfolds a suitably wide block of the folding ruler by 180° (**Fig. 13.8**) and holds it between the test goal (e.g., the wall) and the part of the patient's body that is supposed to touch the test goal (**Fig. 13.9**). If the therapist has estimated incorrectly, he adds or removes the appropriate number of sections until the width of the block equals the distance between the body and the test goal.

Distances of over 3.5 cm are measured using two folding rulers. For this purpose, one ruler is held at a right angle to the test goal (for instance, the wall) (**Fig. 13.10**). The second ruler is angled by 90° and laid against the first ruler so that the angled portion is parallel to the test goal (**Fig. 13.11**). Rulers that lock at a 90° angle are particularly useful for this purpose.

To measure the distance from the test goal, the therapist now lets the angled ruler slide parallel along the second ruler until it reaches the part of the patient's body that is supposed to touch the test goal. When the bent ruler touches this body part, its distance from the test goal can be read on the second ruler (**Fig. 13.12**).

Common metric folding rulers are 3.5 cm wide and, when completely unfolded, 2 m long. If necessary, special 3- or 4-m sized folding rulers that are proportionately wider may also be used.

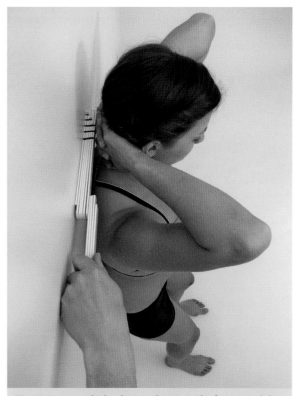

Fig. 13.9 ... equals the distance between the fingers and the wall in this thoracic extension test. In this way, it can be determined that the distance from the test goal in this example is 21 mm.

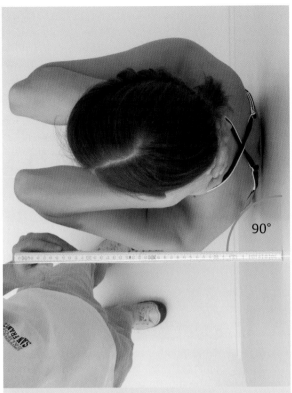

Fig. 13.10 The white ruler is held perpendicular to the wall.

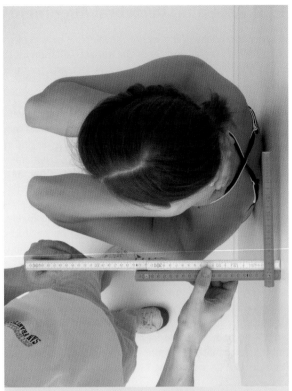

Fig. 13.11 The second blue ruler, angled at 90°, is laid against the white ruler so that the part that is angled by 90° is parallel to the wall.

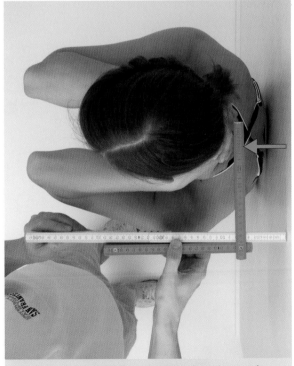

Fig. 13.12 The angled, blue ruler slides along the straight, white ruler toward the body part that is supposed to touch the test goal. When the blue ruler touches this body part, the distance from the test goal can be read on the scale of the white ruler. In this case, the distance is 8 cm.

13.2 Assessing Vertebral Alignment

In order to evaluate the effect of the exercise in Navigator 26 (pp. 177 f.) on the vertebrae, the initial evaluation must be compared with the re-evaluation of vertebral position and mobility after every single exercise.

A simple and quick way to evaluate the position of the vertebrae is to palpate two successive spinous processes in a pincer grip (**Fig. 13.13**). A convenient position to do this in is with your patient sitting on a chair or stool, her forearms resting on the treatment table in front of her, and her forehead resting on her forearms (**Fig. 13.14**), so that her neck muscles relax, and palpation of the spinous processes becomes possible. If no treatment table is available, your patient may instead rest her forehead on her forearms on the back of a suitable chair she is straddling (**Fig. 13.15**).

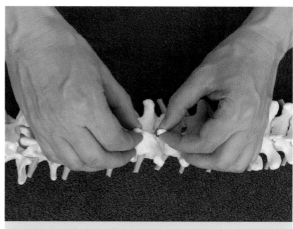

Fig. 13.13 Palpation of the spinous processes.

When the patient is in position, the therapist begins the examination with palpation of the spinous processes of C2 and C3. This is followed, in descending order, by C3 and C4, C4 and C5, etc., as far as L5 and S1. In this process, the therapist marks the spinous processes that deviate to the side with an arrow (**Fig. 13.16**).

Because spinous processes can also be crooked, a deviation of the spinous process of C7 to the right (**Fig. 13.16**), does not prove that the vertebral body of C7 is rotated to the

left. But if the C7 spinous process realigns itself with the other spinous processes (**Fig. 13.17**) after a given exercise, while at the same time the function and symptoms of the C7 area improve, it is highly likely that the vertebral body was, in fact, rotated. Another indication that the C7 vertebral body is rotated to the left is when all the spinous processes below it also deviate to the right (**Fig. 13.18**), because it is unlikely that so many of the subsequent spinous processes would also be crooked.

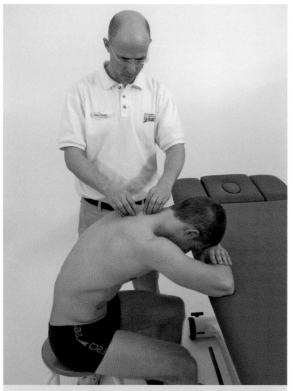

Fig. 13.14 Straddle position on a chair while resting on the treatment table.

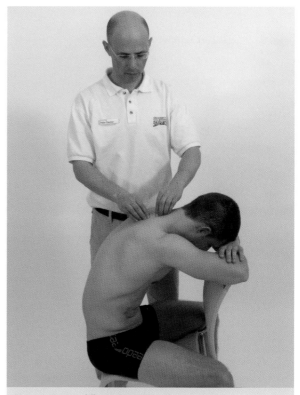

Fig. 13.15 Straddle position on a chair.

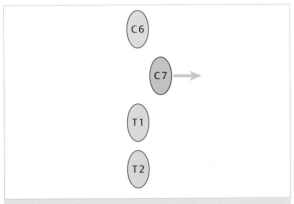

Fig. 13.16 Dorsal view: The spinous process of C7 deviates to the right.

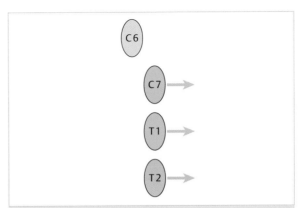

Fig. 13.18 The C7 spinous process, en bloc with all the spinous processes below it, deviates to the right.

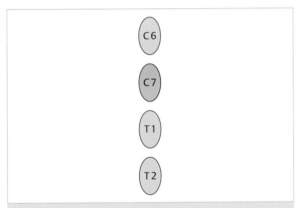

Fig. 13.17 Alignment after repositioning of the C7 spinous process.

13.3 Pain Scale

The following color scale is helpful in documenting your patient's pain on a scale of 0 to 10 (**Fig. 13.19**). It is a so-called visual analog scale, and it is divided into zones 0 to 10 by vertical lines.

Ask your patient to place her finger on the point of the scale that corresponds to her pain, and record the number of the respective zone. So that your patient is not confused or biased by the numbers, you should use the scale without numbers (**Fig. 13.20**).

You can obtain a picture of the long-term development of pain if you note the minimal, maximal, and average pain values at the initial evaluation and compare them with the values "since the last treatment" each time the patient returns for her subsequent appointments.

The immediate effect of an exercise on the pain can be seen by comparing the current pain values immediately before and after the exercise.

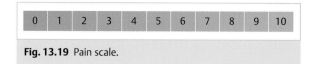

Fig. 13.19 Pain scale.

▶ Where is your pain located on the pain scale?

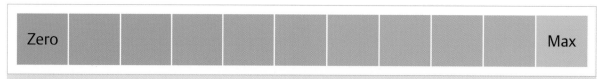

Fig. 13.20 *Zero*, at the far left in the blue zone, means "Absolutely no pain." *Max*, at the far right in the orange zone, means "The worst pain I have ever experienced."

13.4 Exercise Plan for Patients

You can download an exercise plan for patients from www.spinal-fitness.com. You will find this and other downloads under "Information for therapists, trainers, and physicians."

Example of an exercise plan

Fig. 13.21 shows what an exercise plan looks like and how it is used.

Simply check the boxes in front of the exercises your patient should perform, and circle the boxes in front of the tests that she has passed and for which further exercises are not required. This gives you an overview of the tests that have already been done. If necessary, you can indicate the priority of exercises for your patient with A, B, or C, where "A" indicates the highest, "B" a moderate, and "C" a relatively low priority.

If it would be useful for the patient to do more exercises than she can complete in one day, you can also indicate whether an exercise should be done daily (1×/day), or only three times a week (3×/week). Instead of indicating a number of times per week, you can also specify days of the week (e.g., Monday, Wednesday, and Friday) for doing the exercises.

Spinal Fitness Check   www.spinal-fitness.com

Patient: Therapist: Date:

Practice:

☑ Test not passed = exercise   ⬚ Test passed = no need to exercise

Exercises in everyday activities		Extra exercises	

Posture

B ☑ Seated posture with symmetrical foot placement
A ☑ Neutral spinal curvature
  ⬚ Sit...
  ⬚ Stabil...
  ⬚ Balan...
B ☑ Posture-friendly environment
  ⬚ Chair height
  ⬚ Distance between the knees and between the feet
  ⬚ Symmetrical weight distribution when sitting
  ⬚ Stance width
  ⬚ Symmetrical weight distribution when standing
  ⬚ Standing posture with a balanced upper body

> A neutral sitting posture is especially important for this patient and is thus indicated as "A," the highest priority.

Relaxation

  ⬚ Relaxed tongue
  ⬚ Relaxed lower jaw
  ⬚ Relaxed lower lip
  ⬚ Relaxed shoulders
  ⬚ Abdominal breathing

Movement

  ⬚ Changing seated position
  ⬚ Change of position
  ⬚ Dynamic sitting and standing

Coordination

  ⬚ Sitting up
  ⬚ Balance
  ⬚ Arm swing
  ⬚ Hip extension
  ⬚ Eye muscle coordination

Mobility

  ⬚ Chin tuck mobility
daily ☑ Thoracic extension mobility
  ⬚ Back muscle flexibility
  ⬚ Shoulder mobility
  ⬚ Finger flexor flexibility
daily ☑ Arm nerve mobility
Mo, Fr ☑ Rotational mobility
  ⬚
  ⬚
  ⬚
  ⬚ ...ity
daily ⬚ Posterior thigh flexibility
  ⬚ Calf flexibility
  ⬚ Inner thigh flexibility
  ⬚ Hip extension mobility
  ⬚ Anterior thigh flexibility

> Arm nerve mobility should be trained daily, with rotational mobility trained only on Mondays and Fridays (Mo, Fr).

Strength

  ⬚ Abdominal and anterior neck muscle strength
  ⬚ Back muscle strength
  ⬚ Shoulder blade and triceps muscle strength

  ⬚ Endurance

> The test of back muscle strength was passed and the box consequently circled. Back muscle strength training is not necessary.

Simply check the boxes in front of the exercises your patient should perform and circle the boxes in front of the tests that she has passed and for which exercises are not required. This gives you an overview of the tests that have already been done. If necessary, you can indicate the priority of exercises for your patient with A, B, or C, where "A" indicates the highest, "B" a moderate, and "C" a relatively low priority.

Fig. 13.21 Exercise plan for patients.

13.5 Treatment Plan

Advantages of a Treatment Plan

Efficacy and communication

A systematic differentiation of what helps the patient is only possible with a treatment plan—it is an essential tool for finding simple, efficacious solutions. Moreover, the treatment plan provides a sound basis for professional communication with your patient and the referring physician.

For instance, if the distance from the test goal is measured and recorded in the treatment plan, re-evaluation at the next appointment will show how effectively the patient has exercised. This allows for adequate responses by the therapist as follows:

- It becomes evident from the measurements if the patient has exercised successfully. The visible progress and the therapist's praise motivate the patient to continue exercising with commitment.
- If the patient did not exercise enough, the measurements show that she did not fulfill her responsibility. The therapist and patient can then discuss ways of improving compliance with the exercises.
- If, in spite of intensive exercise, the patient has made no progress, it becomes necessary to check whether the exercise is being done correctly. If this is the case, the therapist can see whether the exercise becomes more effective when it is preceded by the manual techniques or exercises that are suggested in the relevant "Troubleshooting" sections.

The treatment plan consists of two pages. On the following pages, you will first find an example of a completed treatment plan (**Fig. 13.22 a, b**) as an example, and then a blank treatment plan (**Fig. 13.22 c, d**), which you may copy for your own use. For everyday use, you can either staple the two pages of the copied blank treatment plan together or print the two pages double-sided. You can also download a copy of the blank treatment plan from www.spinal-fitness.com by selecting "downloads" under "Information for therapists, trainers, and physicians."

PATIENT: Abigail Adams THERAPIST: John Smith Spinal fitness check (www.spinal-fitness.com)

✓ = Exercise/other treatment done, P = plan for next visit, P1 = do first thing next visit, x = stop technique, HEP = add to home exercise program,
↑ = more, ↓ = less, → = no change, // = the effect was, L = left, R = right, + = positive, – = negative

Goal = Improvement of the following findings	1ST TREATMENT Aug 5, 2015	2ND TREATMENT Aug 12, 2015	3RD TREATMENT Aug 19, 2015	4TH TREATMENT	5TH TREATMENT	6TH TREATMENT	7TH TREATMENT	8TH TREATMENT
① With cervical-RL: pain L neck 5–6/10	5 *1/*2 2	4 / 2	2 / 1	/	/	/	/	/
② Cervical resting pain 0–4/10	2 / 0	2 / 0	0 / 0	/	/	/	/	/
③ mg ibuprofen per day	600 /	600 /	200 /	/	/	/	/	/
④		/	/	/	/	/	/	/
⑤		/	/	/	/	/	/	/
⑥		/	/	/	/	/	/	/

*1 = before treatment, *2 = after treatment

"Cervical resting pain 0–4/10" indicates that, on a scale of 0–10, the pain ranges from complete absence of pain (0) to 4.

At the start of the second session, the pain level was at 2.

At the end of the second session, the pain level was at 0.

The pain that was rated at 5 on a pain scale of 0–10 at the start of the first treatment was rated at 1 at the end of the third treatment.

Spinal fitness check								
Posture								
Seated posture with symmetrical foot placement								
Neutral spinal curvature	0% ✓ // ↓ ②	5%	10%	P				
Sitting without side bending or twisting								
Stabilized neutral spinal curvature								
Balanced upper body when seated								
Posture-friendly environment					P = inspect workplace			
Chair height								
Distance between the knees and between the feet								
Symmetrical weight distribution when sitting								
Stance width								
Symmetrical weight distribution when standing								
Standing posture with a balanced upper body								
Relaxation								
Relaxed tongue								
Relaxed lower jaw								
Relaxed lower lip								
Relaxed shoulders								
Abdominal breathing	–	x						
Movement								
Changing seated position								
Change of position								
Dynamic sitting and standing								

At the third session, the patient reported she had managed to sit upright during her day 10% of the time.

The patient never sits upright (0%). The effect (//) of the posture instruction she received during the session (✓) was that the finding ② (cervical resting pain) improved (↓).

The plan, "P", for the fourth session is to recheck the posture.

The plan, "P", for the fifth session is to visit the patient at her workplace in order to check and optimize the ergonomics of the workplace and the patient's posture where necessary.

The patient passed the test because her breathing is naturally abdominal. Therefore "–" for "negative", test passed, is noted. As abdominal breathing exercises are not necessary, "x" is noted for the following treatments to indicate there is no point in working on abdominal breathing.

Sample treatment plan

Fig. 13.22 a Completed example treatment plan, page 1.

Sample treatment plan

	1ST TREATMENT Aug 5, 2015	2ND TREATMENT Aug 12, 2015	3RD TREATMENT Aug 19, 2015	4TH TREATMENT	5TH TREATMENT	6TH TREATMENT	7TH TREATMENT	8TH TREATMENT
Coordination								
Sitting up								
Balance								
Arm swing								
Hip extension								
Eye muscle coordination	+ √ // → ① + ②	X						
Mobility								
Chin tuck mobility	4F √ // ↓ ①+②	3F	2F	P				
Thoracic extension mobility								
Back muscle flexibility								
Shoulder mobility								
Finger flexor flexibility								
Arm nerve mobility	5F // ↑ ①+②	X	L4F R1F √ // → ① ↓ ② 2to1					
Rotational mobility								
Lifting technique								
Hip flexion mobility								
Buttock muscle flexibility								
Leg, back, and cranial nerve mobility								
Posterior thigh flexibility								
Calf flexibility								
Inner thigh flexibility								
Hip extension mobility								
Anterior thigh flexibility								
Strength								
Abdominal and anterior neck muscle strength								
Back muscle strength								
Shoulder blade and triceps muscle strength	20S √ // → ①+②	20 s	35 s	P				
Endurance Minutes per week:	0	30	30	P = 45				
Manual techniques and other types of treatment								
A-P mobilization of the left first rib in the supine position			√ // ↓ ① 2-1	P				
Trial pillow			√	P = How was it?				

During the first session, the eye muscle coordination did not alter the symptoms ① and ②. Due to the lack of response, an "x" was entered to indicate that there would be no point repeating the exercise at the next session.

Arm nerve mobility was not tested until the third session. On the left side, the test goal was missed by 4 finger widths, and on the right side by 1 finger width. The arm nerve mobility exercise did not change the symptom ①; it did, however, lessen the resting pain (②) from 2 to 1 out of 10 on the pain scale. Due to lack of space, the documentation extends into the next field.

At the initial evaluation, the test goal was missed by 4 finger widths (4F). The exercise reduced the symptoms ① and ②.

At the third session, the patient was only short of the test goal by 2 finger widths (2F).

At the end of the third treatment, the therapist planned to test rotational mobility at the next session and noted "p" for "Plan".

Because this exercise exacerbated the symptoms ① and ② during the first treatment, an "x" is noted in the plan for the next session to indicate that it should not be repeated.

At the third session, the patient was able to hold the exercise position for 35 seconds.

The plan for the fourth session is to advise the patient to increase her endurance training to 45 minutes per week.

Because mobilization of the first rib was effective at the third session, the plan is to repeat the mobilization in the fourth session.

At the fourth session, the therapist plans to ask the patient whether the trial pillow at the third session was helpful.

At the first session, the patient was only able to hold the exercise position for 20 seconds. The ability to hold this position had no effect on her symptoms.

b Completed example treatment plan, page 2.

PATIENT: THERAPIST: Spinal fitness check (www.spinal-fitness.com)

✓ = Exercise/other treatment done, P = plan for next visit, P1 = do first thing next visit, X = stop technique, HEP = add to home exercise program, ↑ = more, ↓ = less, → = no change, // = the effect was, L = left, R = right, + = positive, – = negative

*1 = before treatment, *2 = after treatment

Goal = Improvement of the following findings	1ST TREATMENT	2ND TREATMENT	3RD TREATMENT	4TH TREATMENT	5TH TREATMENT	6TH TREATMENT	7TH TREATMENT	8TH TREATMENT
①	*1 / *2							
②								
③								
④								
⑤								
⑥								

Spinal fitness check

Posture

Seated posture with symmetrical foot placement								
Neutral spinal curvature								
Sitting without side bending or twisting								
Stabilized neutral spinal curvature								
Balanced upper body when seated								
Posture-friendly environment								
Chair height								
Distance between the knees and between the feet								
Symmetrical weight distribution when sitting								
Stance width								
Symmetrical weight distribution when standing								
Standing posture with a balanced upper body								

Relaxation

Relaxed tongue								
Relaxed lower jaw								
Relaxed lower lip								
Relaxed shoulders								
Abdominal breathing								

Movement

Changing seated position								
Change of position								
Dynamic sitting and standing								

c Blank treatment plan, page 1.

	1ST TREATMENT	2ND TREATMENT	3RD TREATMENT	4TH TREATMENT	5TH TREATMENT	6TH TREATMENT	7TH TREATMENT	8TH TREATMENT
Coordination								
Sitting up								
Balance								
Arm swing								
Hip extension								
Eye muscle coordination								
Mobility								
Chin tuck mobility								
Thoracic extension mobility								
Back muscle flexibility								
Shoulder mobility								
Finger flexor flexibility								
Arm nerve mobility								
Rotational mobility								
Lifting technique								
Hip flexion mobility								
Buttock muscle flexibility								
Leg, back, and cranial nerve mobility								
Posterior thigh flexibility								
Calf flexibility								
Inner thigh flexibility								
Hip extension mobility								
Anterior thigh flexibility								
Strength								
Abdominal and anterior neck muscle strength								
Back muscle strength								
Shoulder blade and triceps muscle strength								
Endurance Minutes per week:								
Manual techniques and other types of treatment								

d Blank treatment plan, page 2.

13.6 Age and Gender-specific Fitness Curves

Using the following fitness curves (**Fig. 13.23**), you can show your patients how fit they are compared with other persons of the same age and gender. The fitness curves consist of the averages of 1,104 individuals who have gone through all the tests in the book.

The x-axis shows age in 10-year groups. The y-axis shows the percentage of tests in one category (e.g., Posture) that were passed.

The formula with which you can calculate the percentage of tests your patient has passed is: 100 × the number of tests passed divided by the total number of tests. The total number of tests is:

- Posture: 12
- Relaxation: 5
- Movement: 3
- Coordination: 5
- Mobility: 16
- Strength: 3
- Endurance: 90 minutes/week

Examples

>Example 1: Of the total of 12 posture tests, your patient has passed 6: 100 × 6 divided by 12 = 50%. This corresponds approximately to the group of 20–29-year-old women (see the top line chart, "Posture").

Example 2: Of the total of 16 mobility tests, your patient has passed 6: 100 × 6 divided by 16 = 37.5%.

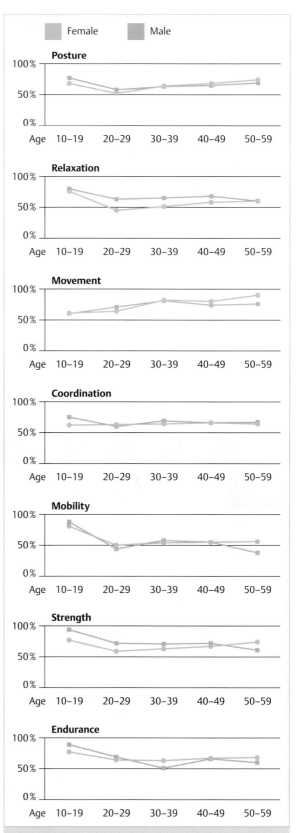

Fig. 13.23 Age- and gender-specific fitness curves.

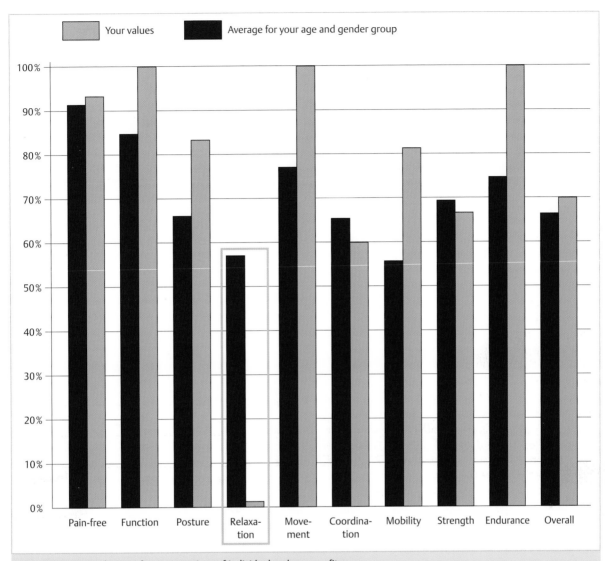

Fig. 13.24 Fitness diagram for a comparison of individual and average fitness.

13.7 Fitness Diagram

As an alternative to the fitness curves, you can also visualize how fit your patient is in comparison to others by means of a bar chart (**Fig. 13.24**). The average values in the bar chart are based on 1,104 persons who have gone through all 45 tests. The bar chart is automatically created when a patient's test results are entered at www.spinalfitness.com in the online check. This appears as a pdf file that may be printed, viewed on screen, or e-mailed. You can create the diagram for your patients and, as you prefer, offer the service for free or for a nominal fee. Alternatively, you can ask your patients to do this for themselves at home, and to bring the printout to the next treatment session.

In communication between the physician and the patient, the diagram makes it easy to point out where the patient's strengths and weaknesses lie. For a physician who has no time to read long reports, a fitness diagram like the example in **Fig. 13.24** makes evident at a glance where any remaining deficits lie and why a follow-up referral for physical therapy is warranted.

13.8 Diagnostic Efficacy

The test results, self-reported pain, and self-reported functional limitations of the 1,104 individuals who underwent all 45 tests in the book were analyzed. Persons with less pain and fewer functional limitations had better test results in all seven fitness categories (from Posture to Endurance) than persons with more pain and a greater number of functional limitations. The difference was statistically significant in most fitness categories, with the exception of coordination. This means that the tests in the other six fitness categories were able to reveal pain- and function-related deficits.

From the clinical point of view, the half of the 1,104 persons who passed a higher percentage of the tests in this book had on average 24% less pain and 6% fewer functional limitations.

13.9 Treatment Efficacy

Therapeutic efficacy is defined as the measure of how effectively symptoms and dysfunctions could be corrected with the exercises in the book.

In a study of 43 patients (Walz 2008), participants reported on the number of regions they were currently experiencing pain in, and the intensity of the pain. Immediately thereafter, they went through all the tests and exercises in this book for the first time (with the exception that endurance was only tested by inquiry, and was not practically tested or trained). At the end, the participants again reported on the location and intensity of any pain. The following changes resulted from the one-time performance of the exercises (**Fig. 13.25**):
- 8% of the painful body regions felt worse.
- 16% of the body regions felt the same.
- 76% of the body regions felt better. In these areas, the pain had decreased by an average of 52%.

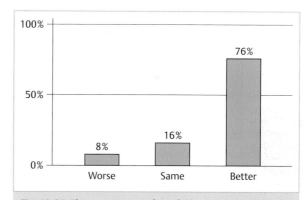

Fig. 13.25 The percentages of painful body regions in which the participants felt more, the same, or less pain after the first performance of the tests and exercises.

References

Adams MA, Hutton WC. The effect of posture on the role of the apophyseal joints in resisting intervertebral compressive forces. J Bone Joint Surg Br 1980; 3: 358–362

Betz U, Grober J, Meurer A. Ist die Thoraxbeweglichkeit bei Patienten mit einem Impingement-Syndrom der Schulter verändert? – Vergleich mit gesunden Probanden. Manuelle Therapie 2005; 9: 2–10

Caro CG, Dumoulin CL, Graham JMR, Parker KH, Souza SP. Secondary flow in the human common carotid artery imaged by MR angiography. J Biomed Eng 1991; 114: 147–153

Dwyer A, Aprill C, Bogduk N. Cervical zygoapophyseal joint pain patterns I: a study in normal volunteers. Spine 1990; 15: 458

Farmer JC, Wisneski RJ. Cervical spine nerve root compression. Spine 1994; 19: 1850–1855

Fischer P. Sitting slumped or upright? Which position is healthier and how can a healthier position be trained? [Article in German.] Manuelle Therapie. 2004; 8: 147–152

Fischer P, Battes S, Axmann D, Engel E. Gender specific differences in posture and back pain at the computer workstation. PhysioScience. 2013; 9(2): 59–64

Fishman LM, Konnoth C, Rozner B. Botulinum neurotoxin type band physical therapy in the treatment of piriformis syndrome. Am J Phys Med Rehabil 2004; 83: 42–50

Hides JA, Jull GA, Richardson CA. Long-term effects of specific stabilization exercises for first episode low back pain. Spine 2001; 26: E243–E248

Jones A, Dean E, Chow C. Comparison of the oxygen cost of breathing exercises and spontaneous breathing in patients with stable obstructive pulmonary disease. Phys Ther 2003; 83: 424–431

Kerr HE, Grant JH, MacBain RN. Some observations on the anatomical short leg in a series of patients presenting themselves for treatment of low back pain. J Am Ostepath Assoc 1943; 42: 437–440

Kim KH, Choi SH, Kim TK, Shin SW, Kim CH, Kim JI. Cervical facet injections in the neck and shoulder pain. J Korean Med Sci 2005; 20: 659–662

Link CS, Nicholson GG, Shaddeau SA, Birch R, Gossman MR. Lumbar curvature in standing and sitting in two types of chairs: relationship of hamstrings and hip flexor muscle length. Phys Ther 1990; 70: 24–31

Little JS, Khalsa PS. Human lumbar spine creep during cyclic and static flexion: creep rate, biomechanics, and facet joint capsule strain. Ann Biomed Eng 2005; 33(3): 391–401

Marshall M, Harrington AC, Steele JR. The effect of work station design on sitting posture in young children. Ergonomics 1995; 38: 1932–1940

Mead J, Loring SH. Analysis of volume displacement and length changes of the diaphragm during breathing. J Appl Physiol Respir Environ Exerc Physiol. 1982; 53(3): 750–755

Nachemson AL. Disc pressure measurement. Spine 1981; 6: 93–97

Petrone MR, Guinn J, Reddin A, Sutlive TG, Flynn TW, Garber WP. The accuracy of the Palpation Meter (PALM) for measuring pelvic crest height difference and leg length discrepancy. J Orthop Sports Phys Ther 2003; 33(6): 319–325

Piper A. Literaturübersicht: Korrelation zwischen lumbalen Rückenschmerzen und dem M. glutaeus maximus. Manuelle Therapie 2005; 9: 65–74

Reinecke SM, Hazard RG, Coleman K. Continuous passive motion in seating: a new strategy against low back pain. J Spinal Disord 1994; 1: 29–35

Rivett DA, Sharples KJ, Milburn PD. Effect of premanipulative tests on vertebral artery and internal carotid artery blood flow: a pilot study. J Manipulative Physiol Ther 1999; 22(6): 368–375

Schäfer M. Erkrankung der Lendenwirbelsäule. Online-PDF-Doktorarbeit 2005

Schüldt K, Ekholm J, Harms-Ringdahl K, Németh G, Arborelius UP. Effects of changes in sitting posture on static neck and shoulder muscle activity. Ergonomics 1986; 12: 1525–1537

Snijders CJ, Hermans PF, Kleinrensink GJ. Functional aspects of cross-legged sitting with special attention to piriformis muscles and sacroiliac joints. Clin Biomech (Bristol, Avon) 2006; 21(2): 116–121

Twomey LT, Taylor JR. Physical Therapy of the Low Back. 2nd ed. New York, NY: Churchill Livingstone: 1994: 415–426

Vickery R. The effect of breathing pattern retraining on performance in competitive cyclists. Online-PDF-Master-Work 2007

Waibel C, Fischer P, Rapp W, Horstmann T. Posture Feedback for Computer Users. Effects on strength, flexibility, well being and activity level. [Artcile in German.] ErgoMed 2013; 2: 32–38

Walz H. The Spinal-Fitness-Check: Its effectiveness as diagnosis and treatment tool, age-dependent development of spinal fitness and gender-specific differences. Bachelor Thesis [in German]. University of Tübingen, Germany; 2008

Wilke HJ, Neef P, Claim M, Hoagland T, Claes LE. New in vivo measurements of pressures in the intervertebral disc in daily life. Spine 1999; 8: 755–762

Yoo W, Yi C, Kim H, Kim M, Myeong S, Choi H. Effects of slump sitting posture on the masticatory, neck, shoulder and trunk muscles associated with work-related musculoskeletal disorders. Physical Therapy Korea 2006; 4: 39–46